BEAR GRYLLS

WITH KAY VAN BEERSUM

FUEL FOR LIFE

BANTAM PRESS

LONDON · TORONTO · SYDNEY · AUCKLAND · JOHANNESBURG

Thank you, Kay, for helping me find an incredible way of making the mega-healthy also mega-delicious – this has been an eye opener and a life changer! And thank you also for enlightening me and my family. You have helped us navigate through the minefield of nutritional research, sifting the truth from the fiction, towards our goal of lean, clean, delicious fuel for life and longevity.

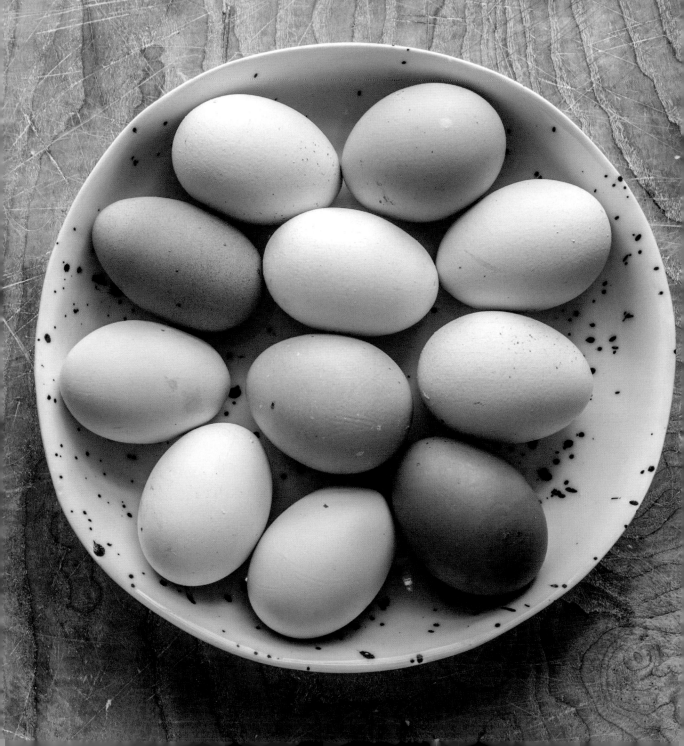

CONTENTS

INTRODUCTION

Here's the deal: I'm fitter, leaner and healthier in my forties than I was at twenty-five, having climbed Everest and served in the British Special Forces. In this book, I'm going to show you how this is possible. And it is simpler than you might imagine.

I trained my backside off in the military and beyond, but it never seemed to lead to the results that I aspired to. And so, even though I had good strength and endurance, and a cast-iron determination to keep going, I didn't ever look like much of an athlete. I just assumed I was the sort of person who could never get a six pack!

I was wrong about that, and the reason I was wrong was because I never thought about what I was eating.

But first, let's briefly rewind.

Smart, life-enhancing nutrition was never on the agenda when I was growing up. I think the reasons were probably both cultural and generational. I was certainly never taught how to eat healthily when I was at school, nor at home when I was a young boy. Meals were often quite hurried affairs, I always remember, and the type of food was very old-school 'English': think lamb chops, potatoes, stewed cabbage, and then for pudding spotted dick and cream. And then, whenever we got hungry between meals, we would race into the kitchen and just make and eat lots of toast with butter and jam.

Then I left school, hit life and joined the army, where nutrition was more about eating as much as you could, as fast as you could, rather than about *what* you were eating. Before I knew it, habits were formed and that was that!

It took a shock to give me the wake-up call that I needed. It was about a year after I'd returned from Everest. I had also now left the military. That was a year of eating too much, not exercising and also writing my first book. I'd just done one of my first ever TV interviews, and I remember watching it back on the screen and realizing how pasty and bloated I was. Not a good look. But still I didn't give it a lot of thought. Then Shara and I got married, didn't have much money, shopped cheap at budget supermarkets, ate pretty badly and witnessed my father die of heart disease. A month later, struggling in so many ways, I was offered the chance to do a TV commercial for Sure deodorant featuring my Everest climb. It felt like a gift from my dad from beyond the grave at a time when I really needed a break. The catch was that I would have to go shirtless! Now that was good motivation. I decided it was time to make a change. I had three months to do it.

I started experimenting boldly. I tried going crazy in the gym. I tried not eating at all. I even remember trying some herbal diet pills I saw advertised on a street corner. I lost a little weight through sheer willpower and (with some clever lighting and camera positioning!) pulled off the advert – just. Soon after that I got more offers for TV and I continued to do whatever I could to get fitter and leaner, again all through willpower and a not very fun approach to food and being disciplined. Trouble was, motivation only got me so far without the right knowledge.

Whatever I did, however much I trained like a monster or adopted the latest Atkins fad, I could never get lean, strong, happy and healthy all at the same time. Whatever I did, whether training harder or eating less, or changing when I ate, or mixing carbs and proteins differently, or eating according to blood type – you name it – nothing worked beyond the occasional short-term blip.

I soon realized that nutrition had to be key to change – otherwise I would have looked much better than I did when I was so fit and strong in the SAS. Nutrition had to be the main factor. But I just didn't understand this murky world of health and nutrition well enough. I knew that I needed to educate myself if I really wanted to see the sort of positive changes that I hoped I could implement.

And so I did. I read widely to expand my nutritional knowledge. I carefully watched the habits of other people who seemed to be getting it right. And as I started to understand a lot more about positive nutrition, about eating for maximum health and longevity, the blinkers of my traditional nutritional beliefs and habits began to come off. Of course I made mistakes along the way, and followed the occasional dead-end, but gradually I developed a way of healthy eating that worked for me. The difference was amazing. I felt great, and I started to look so much better than I did in those early TV days.

But there was still a problem. The food I really enjoyed was the unhealthy stuff. I was still having to be really disciplined and determined to eat right, because it tasted so boring (and it didn't help that I hated vegetables!).

So the next challenge for me was to make the healthy stuff taste incredibly delicious. I didn't want to feel deprived and bored every time I needed to fuel myself. I wanted to get to a stage where I would crave the good stuff because it tasted better than the junk.

Was such a nutritional utopia possible?

I started to seek out amazing recipes that meant I could be enthusiastic about eating healthily and not just see it as a chore. In the beginning, I'd find a single recipe that wasn't mega-fattening or high in sugar, but which tasted awesome, and I'd live off that for a month. Then I would try to improve on it, replace any of the bad ingredients with better ones that I had researched, until we had it where it still tasted amazing but was now 100 per cent health-enhancing. Then I'd find a new recipe – and gradually my store of recipes started to increase. Before long, I found I actually preferred the healthy stuff to the unhealthy stuff – and what is more, the healthy recipes always seemed so much more filling, which meant I would eat much less. Great bang for the buck. I felt fuller, yet I could eat as much as I wanted, it tasted better than the junk food, it made me lean and it got me strong.

Eureka!

That's what this book is about: wholesome, natural food that tastes better than the processed junk many of us have been used to for so long. It is about real food and innovative 'comfort food' recipes which make us feel and look fantastic. We'd be idiots not to give that a go, right?

Of course, it's not just about how we feel and how we look. It's also about our long-term health. In the old days, people used to think that our health was 80 per cent training, 20 per cent nutrition. Now it's widely acknowledged to be the other way round. The vast majority of your health, fitness, wellbeing, mental state, productivity and longevity really is down to what you put in your mouth. When I eat now, I think to myself: 'Is this food really contributing to rejuvenating cells and eliminating toxins? Is it "live" fuel that's really going to help me, or is it going to drain me and put a strain on my system?' I encourage you to ask those questions too, every time you eat. Make it a subliminal habit. With the information in this book, you'll have the tools and the know-how to supply the answers – and then to make the smart choices about how to fuel yourself properly.

When one person recommends someone, I listen. When two people recommend someone, I listen a bit harder. When twenty people recommend someone, I really sit up and take notice. That's what happened with Kay van Beersum, with whom I wrote this book.

Kay looks incredibly healthy, trim and full of life. Before we even spoke, I thought: 'I'm going to listen to this person.'

I'm glad I did. Kay is the most amazing nutritional therapist you'll ever meet. She is incredibly humble, and motivated purely by bringing good health, great nutrition and delicious recipes to everyone. She is the least materialistic person I know – she just wants to make people's lives better, and gets a massive kick out of hearing how their health has improved through the nutritional advice that she's given.

Everything Kay said when we met made sense. She was like a store of all the intel I'd gathered from books and people over the years. When she spoke, everything seemed so simple and logical – like all the best truths in life! It didn't feel like what she was saying would go out of date in a year; it felt like coming home. So much of what I still read and learn about nutrition, day by day, seems to reaffirm what Kay has been saying to me for ages. And when new research comes out, it's so often bang in line with how she's been encouraging me to eat and shop.

Kay has been a great partner in writing this book. She has put in all the long, diligent hours of recipe research – crunching things, throwing them away, re-doing and refining recipes – while my family, friends and I have had the much easier part of testing and tasting them! She is the real hero behind this book and she deserves all the credit. I feel super-privileged to be able to stand beside her in an attempt to get out a message of positive nutrition and life-affirming health that people can adapt for themselves and then stick to for the rest of their lives.

That's the goal! So, welcome to the club and here's to that healthier, leaner, happier, fitter YOU.

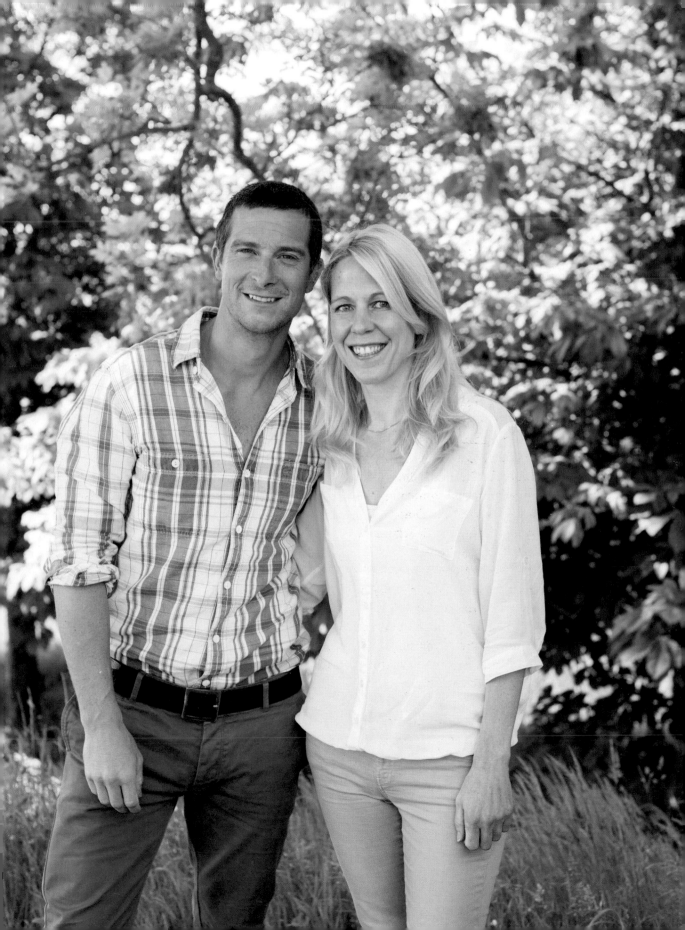

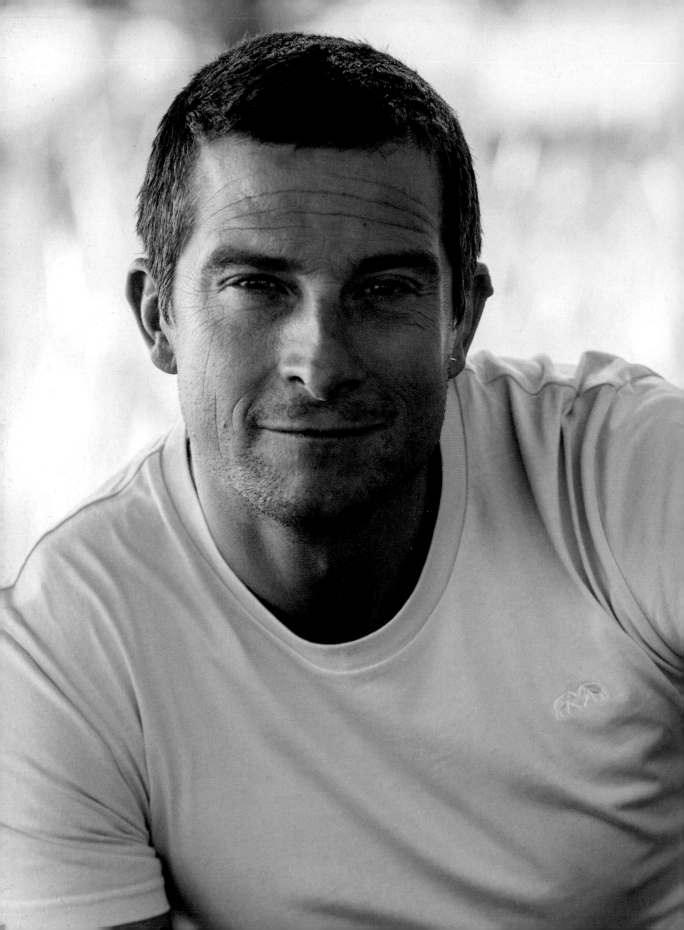

EATING
PRINCIPLES

Without food, we're nothing. And I'm not just talking about when we're in the wild. I'm talking about everyday life.

Food gives us energy. It keeps our brain and other organs functioning. It keeps our heart ticking. It makes our muscles grow and our wounds heal. It keeps our skin, hair and nails healthy and strong. If we don't eat properly, our bodies eventually start to break down and we don't function properly.

But we rarely think about food in this way. People eat for all sorts of reasons – because they're hungry, because they're stressed, because they're bored or because they're in need of a quick energy fix. But how often do we consciously eat for the *real* reason we need food: in order to provide our body with the correct building blocks it depends on to maintain and sustain itself?

Your body is a house (or a car)!

Think of your body as a house. It's built of sturdy bricks, and there's a fireplace that keeps the interior warm. But over time, weather conditions and general use cause wear and tear, both on the interior and the exterior.

Thankfully, there is a constant supply of strong bricks and proper cement to keep the house in tip-top condition, and firewood to keep it warm. With the right supplies, it's easy to keep the wear and tear to a minimum.

Now let's imagine that, instead of using bricks and cement to repair any damage, we choose the easier option and get a big load of sand and dirty water. Instead of firewood, we get a supply of plastic to burn in the fireplace. After all, it's cheaper, looks prettier and is available in abundance.

The sand and water might help you fill in a few cracks. But you soon find that the sand doesn't really stick, and the dirty water just damages the walls. You also find that burning plastic in the fireplace causes smelly smoke to linger everywhere and turns the inside of the house black. But it does kind of keep you warm, so you carry on doing it, as it seems like an easy option, the simplest thing to do . . .

Does that sound to you like a good idea? Didn't think so.

Or think of your body as a brand-new car: shiny, fast and powerful. It requires good fuel and good oil to keep the engine in top condition, and a quality wax to keep it looking great.

But there's some cheaper fuel and oil – easy to get hold of and advertised everywhere as being amazing. And there's a different wax with a prettier tin, so you decide to give that a go.

Time is short – or maybe you're feeling a bit lazy! – and so you leave the car to stand on the driveway or in the garage without much care for it for weeks on end. In no time at all, your car starts to deteriorate. You start to find it needs all sorts of repairs. It doesn't go as fast as once it did, it isn't half as powerful, rust is developing everywhere and things start to break. It doesn't look as good either.

It should be obvious why your house is falling to pieces and is now black with smoke fumes. It should be obvious why your fancy car has started to break down so regularly. But we often fail to understand that our body is no different. By eating unhealthy food, we're not providing it with the bricks it needs to keep it strong and in good condition. We're not giving it the fuel it needs to keep it fast and efficient. We're not giving it the wax it needs to keep it looking awesome.

I want to teach you the secret of eating for longevity and maximum health. And if you think of your body as a house or a car, you'll be halfway there. Now it's a matter of learning how to feed your body the correct nutrients it needs, on a day-to-day basis.

The information in this book will enable you to do this. But first, I want to share with you a few tips I've picked up on my own journey along the path to eating properly.

How can we make healthy food actually taste delicious and satisfying?

If you're anything like me, the question

on your lips is going to be this: how am I going to make healthy food have all the same great flavours that many convenience foods have?

Trust me, it's possible. And here's why: natural foods *do* naturally taste good. We just have to retrain our tastebuds. It doesn't happen in a day, but it's pretty simple and I hope this book will help you speed up the process.

The flavours of unhealthy processed food can be *very* addictive. Flavour enhancers, salt, sugar and fat all seem to trigger in our brains a state of happiness, albeit a temporary one. From a historical point of view, this makes sense.

When I'm hunting for food in the wild, I can't get too obsessed with optimum nutrition. I need to find food that will sustain me, wherever I am and whatever it is. The same was true for our hunter-gatherer ancestors. Food wasn't always readily available for them. They ate whatever they could gather or hunt that day or week. There were inevitably times of starvation. As a result, their bodies evolved to crave those things that sustained them best – foods that gave them the largest calorie intake with the least effort, providing them with instant energy or reserves for bad times to come. Sugar and fat tick these boxes well, so it's hardly surprising that our bodies have learned to crave them, even if they're not that good for us in the long term.

Moreover, sugar, in its many shapes and forms, like salt, is a highly addictive substance. Research shows that sugar may be eight times more addictive than cocaine. A study on salt found that it activates the same parts of the brain as certain narcotics. In my book, that's not good news.

Another problem with salt and sugar is that our tastebuds adjust to our intake. The more you use, the more you need to get the same taste result. If you are a habitual salt user, you'll find that food tastes awfully bland without it.

But we can use this to our advantage. If you reduce your salt or sugar consumption gradually, you will find that your taste for salt and sugar will entirely change. The foods you once loved will seem way too salty or sweet. This change happens quite fast.

So we have some minor addictions to overcome and some retraining to do. In the pages that follow, you'll learn how to replace the bad stuff with more natural alternatives. But I promise you won't have to give up much. In fact, I am about to broaden your options and horizons.

Gain time by spending time
If your life is anything like mine, you're busy. I totally get it when I hear people say they simply don't have the time to cook healthy meals. Long working hours seem to have taken priority over exercise and healthy eating.

But I've found that healthy eating can actually *save* you time. If that sounds confusing, here are two scenarios.

Scenario one
You get into your car after a long day's work. The fish-and-chip shop is on your drive home. You know that when you get home you still have several work emails to write, your bills to pay online and your washing to do. You would love to get some exercise in as well. So, to save time, you drive to the chippie and get a large portion of cod and chips.

After eating the cod and chips you first feel satisfied, then stuffed, and finally rather sluggish. Tiredness sets in fast. Your energy levels drop. So you decide to watch some TV and let the evening pass by until it's time for bed. You tell yourself you'll deal with that backlog of emails, bills, washing and exercise tomorrow . . .

Your evening meal has provided you with a huge influx of calories, an overload of bad fats, salt and carbs – and a lazy attitude!

Scenario two

You get into your car after a long day's work. Your local supermarket is on your drive home. You stop, get some wild salmon steaks, vegetables and sweet potatoes. You grill the salmon with some herbs, boil the vegetables and potato. While the food is cooking, you put your washing on.

Your food is ready in 20 minutes and eaten in 40 minutes. You feel full but not stuffed. Far from being sluggish, you're feeling clear-headed and proud of your amazing cooking skills. You're still fresh enough to attack that backlog of emails and bill payments. An hour later your meal has gone down, your emails and bills are done and you even feel like taking the dog out for a long walk. You still have some time before bed to relax, unwind, watch some TV or read a book.

Your evening meal has provided you with a heap of vitamins, minerals, healthy fats, fibre and protein. It has also left you feeling good, active and energetic. You will even notice the after-effects of this meal in the quality of your sleep, your digestion and in your energy levels when you get up the next morning.

These scenarios are completely realistic. The food you eat can *massively* influence your energy levels. You only need to spend a day in the wild to realize that, but we seem to have forgotten it in everyday life. Food that imbalances our bodies also imbalances our minds. The result is low concentration, aspiration, inspiration, motivation and drive. Who wants to go through life feeling like that?!

Once you get into the routine of cooking healthily every day, the amount of energy you gain will save you so much time. It works for me, and I can't emphasize it enough.

The Shopping Principles section will help you fill up your larder, fridge and freezer so your kitchen will always be equipped for making a quick healthy meal. But no matter where I am, or how busy I am, I always ask myself these four questions before eating:

- ◉ Will eating this food leave me feeling energized or drained?

- ◉ Will eating this food make me feel good about myself or bad about myself?

- ◉ Will eating this food nourish or destroy my body in the short and long run?

- ◉ Will eating this food show respect or carelessness for my body and mind?

The 80:20 rule

I want to live life to the full and I bet you're just the same. To do that, we have to focus on the things we enjoy. For many of us – me included – eating and cooking is part of that enjoyment. In fact, I'd go so far as to say it's one of my passions. I mean, who *doesn't* love the smell of freshly baked bread, or the taste of a cold ice cream on a hot summer's day?

And anyway, life would be pretty boring if we lived by the book all the time. It's healthy to break a few rules every now and again. I like to make that a rule!

I'm hoping to show you that enjoying food doesn't have to mean focusing on fattening, sugar-laden things. That you can get just as much enjoyment from freshly prepared, healthy meals and snacks. In fact, I want to go one further, and show you that the enjoyment you get from this kind of food lasts much longer than the temporary kick you get from an unhealthy snack. That healthy food helps to enhance you mentally and physically, that it improves your mood and your life in the long run, and that it nourishes your body, your mind and your spirit.

But let's face facts: we are all human, and sometimes we like to indulge and not think about the long-term consequences. We all need a mental break from being disciplined and strong. Think of all those women on the *Titanic* who passed on the dessert trolley!

So having the odd break is totally OK, and it's why I stick to an 80:20 rule. For 80 per cent of the time I choose to eat a diet that is rich in good-quality fresh fruits, vegetables, good fats, proteins and unrefined carbohydrates – all the stuff that you're going to read about in the following pages.

And for 20 per cent of the time – if I'm out with friends, having a barbecue, at a birthday party or simply because I want to – I eat whatever I fancy. This means that although my food choices have become super-healthy, I will still occasionally tuck into a burger and chips

and cheesecake. I don't see this as a problem. In fact, Tim Ferriss, the author and fitness guru who conducted countless experiments on himself for his nutritional studies, goes so far as to say that a 'cheat day' per week is vital! He proved it actually kick-started his metabolism for the week ahead, and positively impacted both his health and his fitness goals of maintaining lean muscle. Awesome all round, Tim. Good work!

So yes, I love and look forward to a good cheat day or meal (although so many of the recipes in this book are so darned delicious, cheat meals no longer quite have the appeal they did when the gulf between the taste of healthy food and junk food was much bigger! Ironically, I promise you my chocolate cheesecake is way tastier than any unhealthy one in a restaurant, but there we go!).

Practically speaking, this 80:20 'cheating' works out as either one cheat *day* per week, or a couple of cheat *meals* spread over the week, depending on what's going on or where I am. I aim to stay disciplined with this routine even on holiday. It actually isn't that hard after a while, and the goal of this book is to make the healthy food as delicious, if not more so, than the junk! Then it becomes really easy to keep it going.

So a cheat day, or a couple of cheat meals, are always a treat to me – they are never 'routine' – and often they actually fire up my motivation for that clean, lean week ahead of me.

A positive word of warning, though: you might find that once you start eating more of the healthy stuff, your body will no longer like it when you eat the bad stuff. It could be that all the things you *used* to eat make you feel uncomfortable, give you bad digestion or make you feel very tired or sluggish. It's a good sign that your body is tuning up and that it recognizes that the trash food isn't helping you. Use that feeling as motivation for the clean, lean week ahead – for the positive 80 per cent coming up.

Follow our key steps and some of those nagging health symptoms you thought were part of you may disappear like snow in the sun. This happened to me and I have seen it happen to so many of the crew we film with, as well as to our families. Eating lean, clean and natural is becoming a positive way of life for so many in our BG world of adventure,

and I am so proud of that. We have learned these key nutrition lessons together, and we are all better, stronger and healthier for it! (It always makes me smile when I see kale chips and chocolate protein bombs waiting for us in the crew base camps when I arrive on location in some jungle somewhere!)

50:50

If the 80:20 rule sounds too tough to begin with, that's OK too. It's up to *you* to decide how fast you want to go.

So, if you feel you are carrying quite a bit of extra weight, you rarely exercise and most of your meals are ready meals or takeaways, you may want to start with

KAY SAYS...

Our bodies constantly strive to be in a state of balance. This balance is called 'homeostasis'. Because of the daily stress we endure, the toxins we are exposed to and the unhealthy food we eat, maintaining homeostasis is quite a hard task! In order to cope, our bodies make subtle changes. For example, our liver may have to work a little harder to deal with excess alcohol. Our bones and joints may have to make some adjustments to be able to carry the extra pounds around our waist and hips. Our bowels will have to work super-hard to digest some of the heavy, unhealthy foods we often eat and our hearts have to become more efficient at pumping blood around arteries that are slowly clogging up.

This starts to cause noticeable wear and tear. You may start waking up with aching joints. You may feel bloated or start suffering from acid reflux after a meal. Your skin may lose some of its shine, and you may have dark

circles under your eyes more often than not. We become so accustomed to our bodies constantly coping and adjusting that we consider most of these symptoms as normal.

Of course, our bodies *do* deteriorate with time, but to a large degree we can control how quickly this happens. Many of the subtle aches and pains, digestive issues, skin problems or reduced energy we experience as time passes are signs that we are doing something wrong. Peptic ulcers, type 2 diabetes, gout, heart disease and arthritis are often self-inflicted through diet and lifestyle. The foods we gradually ask you to cut out in this book can often be the culprit. People who eliminate white bread and other white flour products may find that re-introducing these foods will give them bad bloating and tiredness, whereas once they may have been part of their staple diet and the bloating may have seemed normal.

a 50:50 approach. Incorporate healthy meals 50 per cent of the time and stick with your old habits for the other 50. Your newfound energy levels during those times when you follow the new regime will soon encourage you to up the ratio.

If you consider yourself fairly healthy but don't quite know all the facts about healthy eating or know how to prepare all your meals, start with a 70:30 approach. It won't take you more than a few weeks to achieve the aim of 80:20.

However, I do feel it is always good to dream big and go big! Small goals rarely lead us anywhere significant – and if it was me and I wanted to see change and get lean, I would go for it and make those changes positive and big. 80:20 really isn't too extreme or crazy. All my family and kids manage it without much drama; and even if you aim for it but initially fall a little short, at least you are now making some real headway towards a healthier, leaner you.

The eight-week programme at the end of the book is suitable for everybody. It allows you to take all the necessary steps at your own pace and in your own time. But before you embark on any of this, it's important you know *why* you're doing it. The next section – 'The Bear Facts' – will give you the low-down on the good, the bad and the ugly of all the foods we're used to eating . . .

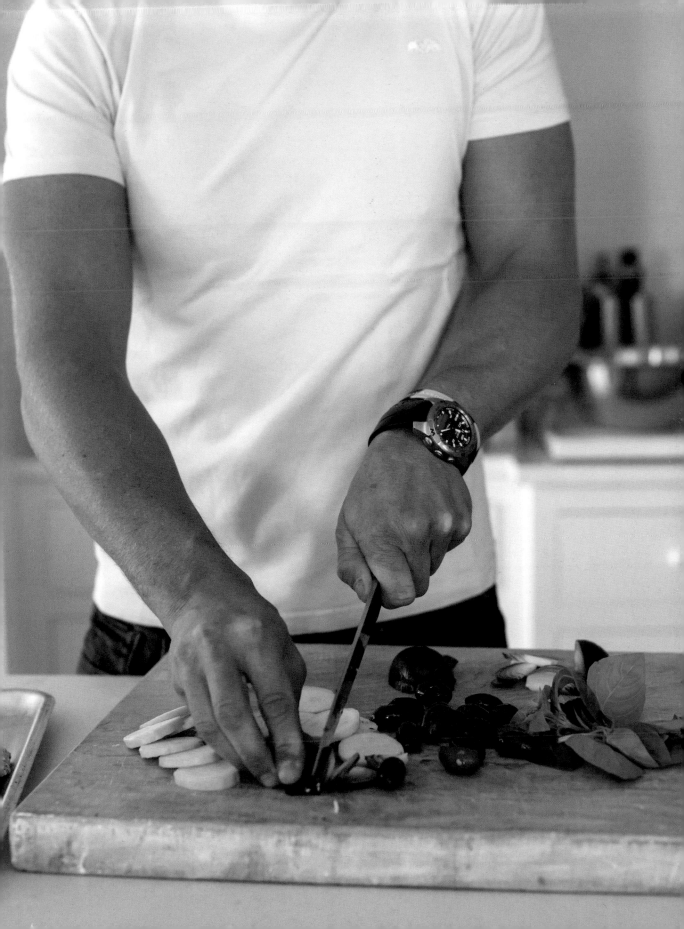

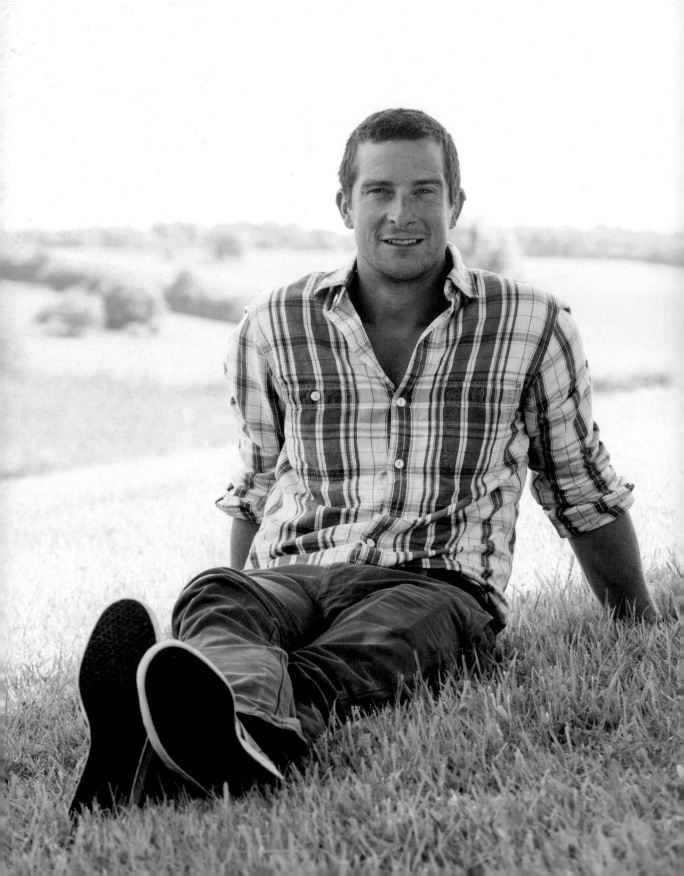

THE
BEAR
FACTS

CALORIES

First off, what is a calorie?

The word was first defined in the nineteenth century as a unit of measurement, particularly in relation to the study of heat and energy in machines. One calorie is the quantity of energy needed to raise the temperature of 1kg of water by 1°C. As time went by, the calorie started to be used as a measurement of energy in the human body, and it became a fashionable tool for weight loss.

I personally don't believe in counting calories. That's not because eating fewer calories can't help you to lose weight. It can. But there's a flaw: not all calories are the same.

We can divide calories into two types: nutritional calories and empty calories. Empty calories do not contribute to health, whereas nutritional calories do.

We need certain vitamins, minerals, proteins, fats and carbs for our bodies to function properly, to prevent us from getting ill and to keep us feeling fit, full of energy and ready for anything. Some foods – let's call them nutritious foods – contain a whole host of these good things. Other foods – let's call them empty foods – are devoid of the good stuff. But nutritious foods and empty foods can contain the same number of calories.

To show you what I mean, let's imagine we eat a total of 380 calories in snacks, but in two different ways: the first eating empty foods, the second eating nutritious foods.

EMPTY FOODS

1 bag of ready salted crisps, 230 calories
1 thick slice of white toast, 79 calories
1 digestive biscuit, 71 calories

Total: 380 calories

Nutritional content: high in unhealthy fats, salt, sugar and additives. Devoid of vitamins and minerals

Effect on health: detrimental to blood-sugar balance, hormone balance, heart health, digestion, energy levels, brain function, mood, skin, hair and nails

NUTRITIOUS FOODS

½ avocado, sea salt and pepper, 160 calories
40g hummus with ½ sliced red pepper, 70 calories
3 dates and 3 walnuts, 150 calories

Total: 380 calories

Nutritional content: rich in fibre, healthy fats, protein, minerals and vitamins

Effect on health: awesome for blood-sugar balance, hormone balance, heart health, digestion, energy levels, brain function, mood, skin, hair and nails

Empty foods can really knock you out of the game. And because they don't provide you with anything the body needs, you often end up craving more. Your body can't speak to you in words, so if it needs more protein, for example, it sends signals to your brain asking for more food, any food, hoping you pick the right stuff. You know how one piece of toast never seems to be enough? The same goes for crisps and biscuits. They provide nothing but empty calories. But I doubt you'd still feel hungry after eating an entire avocado.

Choose quality over quantity – always!
Food is fuel. If you fill your car with bad fuel, you may have a full tank but it won't run as nicely or last as long. The same goes for the food that you eat. Fill up on bad fuel and empty calories and you'll eventually start to feel run down and low in energy, and your health deteriorates. Fill up on decent fuel – by which I mean nutritious foods – and you'll feel great.

Food should be fun!
Counting calories can also really take the fun out of eating. So many factors have to be taken into consideration. How long have you slept? How much exercise have you done? Did you walk or drive to the supermarket? Should you starve yourself tomorrow to make up for bad behaviour today?

Despite an abundance of food, in the West we are actually doing a really good job of becoming quite malnourished. This isn't because we aren't eating enough, but because we aren't eating the right foods. It might sound crazy that we can suffer from vitamin or mineral deficiencies considering the amount of food available to us, but it does happen. There's a name for being overweight but undernourished: type B malnutrition. Don't let it happen to you.

I see a lot of people obsessing over how many calories they've burned when they do a workout. To be honest, I can't imagine having to do maths each time I eat or exercise. What a chore! I'd much rather have a relaxed lifestyle knowing that all the foods I eat do good to my body. And now I know that calorie-counting sidesteps the real issues behind good nutrition, I'm happy to swap the calculator for a plate of real food.

Losing weight the right way
A lot of people start counting calories if they want to lose excess weight. They need to be careful.

Excess toxins are stored in fat. When you burn that fat up, these toxins can start to circulate through your body. It's the job of your liver and kidneys to get rid of them. But your liver and kidneys require a lot of vitamins and minerals to function properly. If you lose weight by eating mostly empty calories, they won't have the supply of vitamins and minerals to do their job properly. You'll probably end up feeling sluggish and tired, with dark circles under your eyes. You think that by losing weight you're going to be ready for anything the world throws at you. But you're not.

If you lose weight using nutrient-dense calories, however, your liver and kidneys should function well and will be able to deal with the excess toxins. Chances are you'll feel fit, slim, healthy and energetic at the same time. For me, when I know I have to be at the top of my game, that's the holy grail.

PROTEIN

You've probably seen me eat some pretty grim foods in my search for life-giving protein. Don't worry: live witchetty grubs aren't on the menu today. But protein is just as important a food in everyday life as it is in the wild, so we need to think carefully about what it is and where we get it from.

I'll come clean. If you'd asked me a few years ago what protein is, how the body uses it and what foods are a good source of protein, I don't think I'd have given you a very good answer. I'd probably have said that it's mostly used to build muscle mass, and that it's found in meat and eggs. Why? Because I'd seen loads of my more muscular buddies eating piles of chicken or four-egg omelettes after their weightlifting sessions in the gym, or scoffing massive steaks after a day of rugby or football. That never quite worked for me, though, and here's why: although my answer wasn't completely off, it's only the tip of the iceberg.

Proteins aren't just there to help you build muscle, and they certainly don't only come from meat and eggs. They're far more fundamental than that. They are the primary building blocks of all plant and animal life. Without proteins, life wouldn't exist. Sure, our muscles are made from protein, but so are parts of our skin, bones, hair, nails, eyes, organs, glands and other tissues. Not to mention that our hormones, immune cells, neurotransmitters, enzymes and blood cells mainly consist of protein. Together with water, protein is the most abundant substance in our body.

So: all in all, pretty important.

What are proteins made of?

Proteins are made of tiny building blocks called amino acids. Scientists are divided about the exact number of amino acids, but there are about twenty commonly known ones. Think of them as different-coloured Lego blocks. By clicking blocks together, you could make a vast number of different structures. In the same way, our body can make thousands of different proteins – all the protein it needs – from just these twenty amino acids.

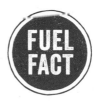

FUEL FACT

The word protein comes from the Greek word protos which means 'first'. Makes sense: proteins are the first building block the body needs for growth, repair, proper immune function, hormone balance, reproduction, digestive function, brain function and muscle function.

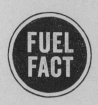

Of these twenty, our body can manufacture eleven without any outside help. We need to get the remaining nine from our food. The nine amino acids that we cannot manufacture ourselves are called the 'essential' amino acids. Our body breaks down the protein that we eat into amino acids, then creates new proteins out of them.

Meat, eggs and fish contain all nine essential amino acids. But so do certain plant foods, such as: **quinoa**, **hemp**, **amaranth**, **buckwheat**, **chia seeds**, **soya** and some **sea vegetables.**

In addition, there is a long list of plant foods that contain not all but *many* of the essential amino acids, such as: **nuts**, **seeds**, **beans** and **pulses**, **avocado**, common vegetables such as **broccoli**, **spinach**, **kale**, **sweet potato**, grains such as **oats**, **rice** and **millet**, **sprouts** and **mushrooms**.

In fact, *all* plant foods will contain *some* of the nine essential amino acids. You just have to combine several of them to get all nine in your diet. The good news is, that's pretty easy. You could mix oats with seeds and nuts. You could make a vegetable curry with sweet potato, spinach and lentils. You could add some spirulina and avocado to your morning smoothie. All these combinations should provide you with enough amino acids to make the proteins your body needs. And remember, you don't need to get all nine in each meal.

If it sounds simple, that's because it is: it just boils down to eating a good variety of healthy, natural foods.

Plant versus animal protein

In the wild, there are often two ways to do things: the hard way and the easy way. Most of the time, the smart choice is to take the easy way. It frees up precious energy and time.

It's the same with diet, and especially proteins. Imagine eating a rare steak. First you have to cut it into small pieces. Then you have to chew it thoroughly before you can swallow it. But the process of breaking the food down has hardly even begun. Your stomach and bowels have to work extra hard to break down this partly chewed piece of meat so that the proteins can be extracted from it. And if your digestion doesn't work 100 per cent – which is often the case for people who live a stressful Western lifestyle – it can be extremely hard work. The bottom line is that meat takes a long time and a lot of energy to digest.

Plant proteins are different. They tend to be a lot easier to digest. Take a ripe avocado. Just the process of eating it is easy – you can blend it in a smoothie, spoon it straight from the skin or make an avocado spread. And once it's inside you, things are simpler too. Compared to a piece of steak, your body only has to do half the work to extract the protein. *Plant proteins come in a naturally easy-to-digest form.* This may be one of the reasons why people on a plant-based diet generally seem to live longer and healthier lives – they are saving so much energy by not having to break down all the meat most of us eat.

As you'll read elsewhere in this book, meat can have its place in a healthy diet. But the main message is that protein is in almost all the plant-based foods we eat every day. We don't *need* meat with every meal, and we certainly don't need to worry about not getting sufficient protein if we don't eat meat daily. It's virtually impossible to become protein-deficient on a well-balanced plant-based diet.

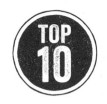

Plant Protein
Sources
hemp seeds
quinoa
avocado
nuts
peas
spinach
chickpeas
broccoli
oats
buckwheat flour

How much protein do we need?

It is recommended that you eat just under 0.9g of protein per 1kg of body weight. But that's just a rule of thumb. The actual amount you need differs from person to person and depends on several factors, such as your age, your weight, your body size and type, whether you're pregnant, your current state of health and, of course, how much exercise you do. Someone who exercises daily will need more protein than someone who sits on the sofa playing video games all day. The recipes in this book are well balanced and should provide you with a healthy amount. But if you really want to go into detail, there are several apps available for your phone which will calculate your recommended protein intake.

However, you should remember this: too much protein can be damaging. Firstly, too much of *any* kind of food will lead to weight gain. Secondly, when we digest protein – especially animal protein – the process produces waste products. Our kidneys have to work hard to filter out these waste products, and this puts an extra burden on them. This is another good reason for reducing your overall meat intake and trying to get more of your protein from plant foods.

Where do protein powders fit in?

First things first: when I say protein powders, I don't mean those heavily flavoured, highly sweetened ones stuffed full of additives to make them taste 'nicer'. I'm talking about natural, unprocessed protein powders. My three favourites are hemp, rice and pea protein.

Hemp protein – contains healthy fats such as omega-3, as well as good amounts of fibre for healthy digestion. It is green in colour and some people find the taste a bit overpowering. To dip your toe in the water, add a tablespoon to a smoothie, or try the amazing hemp Protein Bombs on pages 171, 172. You'll barely taste the hemp, but the balls are delicious and will give you tons of energy.

Rice protein – much milder in flavour and can be added to smoothies in larger quantities without overpowering the taste. Opt for organic sprouted brown rice protein for the best quality.

Pea protein – tastes a little like . . . peas! It works well in savoury dishes like blended soups. Don't heat the powder – add it only after you've finished cooking.

When it comes to protein powders we should always aim for vegan, non-wheat, non-dairy sources. The whey-protein argument continues among athletes. Whey protein has its merits and downsides and the discussion will go on, but my research leads me and millions of others to believe it is always smarter for long-term health to find the best protein from a plant-based source, so I almost always use a vegan protein powder.

I am not militantly against whey, and I do occasionally use it when travelling, but it is not my preferred choice. If you do want to use whey, pick the ones with the least added sugar (sweetened with stevia is OK) and the fewest artificial flavours.

SUGARS & CARBOHYDRATES

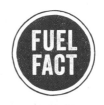

Many foods – fruits, vegetables, beans, grains, pasta, bread, potatoes, cakes and sweets – contain carbohydrates. But not all carbohydrates are the same. They can roughly be divided into two main groups: unrefined carbohydrates and refined carbohydrates.

Unrefined carbohydrates

When we eat carbohydrates, our body breaks them down into smaller units of glucose. Glucose is the main energy source for our muscles and brain. Some carbohydrates are broken down into glucose molecules very quickly. Others are broken down slowly.

Generally speaking, the more unrefined and unprocessed a product is, the more fibre it contains and the more time the body needs to break it down. This is a good thing, and here's why.

Fibre is beneficial in many ways. It helps to make us feel fuller for longer. It helps to slow down the release of glucose into our blood. This in turn helps to balance our blood sugar and energy levels. Fibre attracts water, which bulks up our stool and makes it easier to go to the loo. It also stimulates the healthy bacteria in our gut, which help us digest our food properly and keep our immunity strong.

We need to eat a minimum of 30g of fibre a day. Lots of people think that brown bread and bran are the best ways to get your daily fix – but they're not, because they contain very few other nutrients. It's much better to get your fibre from natural, unrefined plant foods which are stuffed full of it: think vegetables such as **broccoli**, **cabbage**, **kale**, **peas**, **Brussels sprouts**, **spinach**, **parsnips**, wholefoods such as **brown rice**, **quinoa**, **seeds**, **nuts**, **oats**, **beans** and **pulses**.

Potatoes vs sweet potatoes

Potatoes contain very little fibre but are high in starch. For this reason, they tend to be digested quickly into glucose and can cause a massive spike in our blood-sugar levels. This does a real number on our energy levels and general health. (They are also part of the nightshade family, to which many people react badly.)

Sweet potatoes, despite their name, belong to a different family. They contain more fibre, have less of an impact on our blood-sugar levels and are a great source of vitamin A. They also taste amazing!

I eat sweet potatoes in moderation, but certainly try to choose them over ordinary potatoes. It's a simple thing, but it has helped my health massively. (Though you might occasionally see me with a bowl of chips on cheat days!)

SOME HEALTHY SUGAR SUBSTITUTES

Molasses – a treacle-like substance with a very rich flavour. Although it's a by-product of making white sugar from sugar cane, it is relatively rich in vitamins and minerals such as B6 and iron.

Coconut sugar and **jaggery** – this is made from the sap tapped from palms. It contains fibre and a variety of valuable vitamins and minerals. It has less of an impact on blood-sugar levels than white sugar.

Xylitol – a low-calorie sweetener made from plant fibres. It's great for diabetics, but can cause an upset stomach if consumed in large quantities.

Stevia – a natural plant sweetener that does not affect your blood sugar or your teeth. The taste varies depending on the brand, so experimentation is required.

Refined carbohydrates

Refined carbohydrates are usually heavily processed. This means that most of the fibre and other rough bits are removed, but also lots of vitamins and minerals. In fact, over twenty valuable nutrients may be removed in the refining process. Good examples of this are all white-flour products (including white pasta) and white rice.

Refined carbohydrates are very easily and quickly broken down into glucose. Even the saliva in our mouths can do this, so theoretically you could absorb glucose from your diet without even swallowing your food.

Refined carbs don't do us much good. As the fibre has been removed, they can clog up the bowels. The removed fibre also contains lots of valuable nutrients, such as B vitamins, vitamin E and magnesium. When you eat a refined carbohydrate, you are eating a food almost entirely devoid of nutrients. And since they are digested so quickly and easily, they often leave us hungry for more.

Sugar

Sugar is a carbohydrate and is found in almost every processed food you can buy. Don't expect only to find it in sweet-tasting foods such as biscuits and chocolate. You'll find it in crisps, ready meals and sauces, canned soups, bread, breakfast cereals and processed meat, to name a few. Start checking ingredient labels for their total sugar content. About 4 grams of sugar equals a full teaspoon. Fruit drinks especially contain loads (don't be fooled by the amount of sugar per 100ml – we usually drink 250ml, if not more). You may be very surprised to find how many teaspoons of sugar you consume daily.

Trouble is, sugar isn't always labelled as sugar. There are so many hidden names for it, some of which actually sound quite healthy, for example: 'evaporated cane juice', 'barley malt syrup', 'beet sugar', 'corn sweetener', 'corn syrup', 'white grape juice concentrate'. Other substances sound less healthy, and are equally bad: 'hydrogenated starch hydrosylate', 'dextrose', 'disaccharide', 'lactose', 'HFCS', 'liquid maltodextrin'.

Our brains are programmed to like sugar. It's our easiest energy source and in times of scarcity it's the stuff that keeps us going. A survival food, nothing more, nothing less.

So you might think I'd be a fan of it. Sure, in a survival situation I'd take sugar over no food at all. But in everyday life I've learned to be careful of it.

Whenever we eat sugar – or indeed any carbohydrate – the amount of glucose in our blood increases. To be able to use this glucose, our pancreas releases a hormone called insulin. Insulin helps take the glucose out of our bloodstream and into our cells, where it can be used. That's why you get a burst of energy after eating something sweet.

If the glucose isn't used up, it is stored in the muscles and liver for later use. But there's a limited amount of storage space, so if we eat way more than we use, our body converts the glucose into fat for long-term storage. This is why sugar can make us fat.

I have found it nearly impossible to cut out carbohydrates and sugar completely. But I now limit my intake to *unrefined* carbohydrates and natural sugars only. This means sugars from fruits or sugar sources that are as unprocessed as possible. My three favourite sweeteners are **stevia**, **dates** and **maple syrup**.

Stevia

Stevia is a sweetener made from a beautiful green plant. It has been used as a natural sweetener in South America for centuries. As with many 'novel' foods, it took years for stevia to be allowed as a sugar substitute in Europe and North America, but it's now available in most major supermarkets and health shops.

Stevia contains virtually no calories. It doesn't raise blood-sugar levels. It's suitable for diabetics. It doesn't harm your teeth – in fact, it can help to reduce dental plaque. And it can be used for loads of cooking purposes.

It took me a little while to get used to stevia. The important thing is not to use too much, as this may make your food *too* sweet, or even slightly bitter. It might seem pricey at first, but once you realize how little you need in a recipe, you'll see that it's not expensive at all.

A word of warning: not all brands of stevia are the same. Some are a mixture of stevia with an artificial sweetener or even plain old sugar – which entirely defeats the purpose of using it in the first place. They also taste different – there are some good, some better and some awful-tasting ones out

SOME HEALTHY SUGAR SUBSTITUTES

Dates – high in fibre, vitamins and minerals, but also high in natural fruit sugars. Excellent in baking, but consume in moderation.

Maple syrup – naturally super-sweet so you won't need much to create a sweet flavour. Tapped from the maple tree, it contains valuable antioxidants, vitamins and minerals.

Lucuma powder - this super-healthy powder is made from the fruits of the lucuma tree. It has a sweet, caramel-like taste and is rich in fibre, antioxidants, vitamins and minerals. A great addition to drinks, smoothies or deserts.

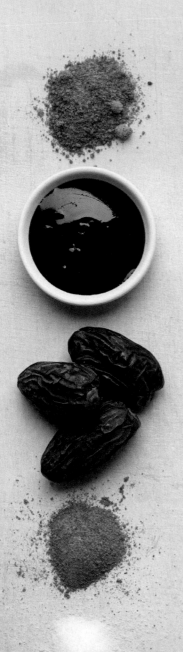

there. Don't give up if you don't like the taste of the first brand you try.

To start incorporating stevia into your diet, use it instead of sugar to sweeten your tea, coffee or hot chocolate. Sprinkle it over tart fruit. Use it to make sugar-free lemonade (page 230). And experiment with it in baking. You'll soon be a convert, just like me.

Dates

Dates are an awesome fruit and a brilliant natural sweetener. They are high in natural fruit sugars. So, unlike stevia, they *do* have an effect on our blood sugar and *can* contribute to weight gain if you eat too many of them. But dates are still far better for us than refined sugar because they are an excellent source of fibre, vitamins and minerals. They provide a great replacement for white sugar in making sweet treats.

The sugars in dates are very quickly absorbed into the body. This makes them an awesome workout fuel – much better than sugary drinks or snacks because they have so many other health benefits.

Maple syrup

I love maple syrup: it comes straight from the maple tree and tastes awesome. It also packs a decent amount of antioxidants, vitamins and minerals. But I'd be lying if I said it was super-healthy. It's very sugary, so you shouldn't have too much.

Good-quality maple syrup is expensive, which is another reason why you might want to only use it sparingly. It gives a great flavour and this means you don't have to resort to loads of white sugar.

Make sure you keep it in the fridge once you've opened it, or it can go mouldy.

Other sweeteners

There are all sorts of chemical sweeteners out there. I'm not a fan. There is plenty of evidence that they can do us harm in the long run. In any case, I'd rather not wait to find out and have stopped using them altogether.

There are, however, a few other healthier sweeteners I'd be happy to use. They are: **molasses**, **coconut**, **sugar**, **jaggery** and **xylitol**.

FAT

I remember the days when we were made to believe that all fat was bad. Low-fat products were – and often still are – presented as the magic solution to weight loss. And like lots of people, I used to think that eating a low-fat version of something meant it had fewer calories, which in turn meant I could eat twice as much of it! (In reality, the low-fat version usually meant more sugar and artificial flavours in an attempt – usually unsuccessful – to make it taste as good as the full-fat version.)

But we need to get past the notion that all fat is bad. Sugar and carbohydrates can do you *way* more harm *and* make you fat. Even if you were to cut out *all* the fat in your diet, you could still gain weight by eating carbohydrates only. More to the point, cutting out all the fat from your diet could do your body some serious harm.

We *need* fat. Not only does it provide a highly concentrated form of energy, it's essential to human life. Every cell in our body is surrounded by a double layer of fat molecules. Without these molecules, our cells would simply fall apart. Fats are needed to make all sorts of hormones in our body. A layer of fat protects our bodies and organs, and it insulates us. Fats transport certain important vitamins around the body, such as vitamins A, D, E and K (so-called 'fat-soluble' vitamins). Not to mention that fats keep our brains functioning at optimal levels. They are crucial for survival.

But there are good fats and bad fats. The important thing is to distinguish between the two. We'll start with the bad.

Bad fats

Hydrogenated oils, partially hydrogenated oils and trans-fats
These are mostly chemically manufactured fats. The human body cannot use or process them, and they can cause a *lot* of serious damage to your health. They contribute to inflammation and cellular damage, and they raise bad cholesterol. If you see them listed on a food label, avoid them like the plague! You can find them in biscuits, cakes, crisps, frozen meals, milky hot drinks, some vegetable spreads and other processed foods. Most UK supermarkets have eliminated these types of fats from their own product lines, but make sure to read the labels of non-supermarket-brand items carefully.

Fat in fried foods
Fat heated to high temperatures is bad news. It creates 'free radicals'. In the cholesterol chapter, you'll learn that these are real bad guys. Fried foods are covered in free-radical-laden oil. You should have them in minimal amounts on 'cheat days' only. A bag of crisps or a bowl of chips on occasion won't kill you, but be smart as to how frequently you eat these.

Saturated fats from factory-farmed animals and dairy
The latest research seems to suggest that saturated fat isn't necessarily bad for us, in moderation. It's a great energy source and can be healthy in small amounts. However, you want to avoid saturated fat from dairy and factory-farmed meat. A high intake of such fats can put a burden on the liver and increase the production of 'bad' cholesterol (see page 38). And don't forget that saturated fats are hard, which means they can harden our cell walls if we eat too much of them.

The best way to get your saturated-fat intake is from plant sources, such as **nuts**, **seeds** and **avocados**, and in small quantities from **lean organic** or **wild meat** and **fish**. But moderation is key.

Pure or refined vegetable oils
We're talking canola oil, rapeseed oil, rice-bran oil,

soya-bean oil, sunflower oil, safflower oil, peanut oil and pure or light olive oil.

Don't be fooled by the term 'pure' or 'vegetable'. These oils are heavily processed and far from pure. They are transparent, odourless and tasteless because they have gone through extensive chemical processes using solvents, high heat and bleaching agents to extract the oil from the base product – for example, a sunflower seed. None of the health benefits of the actual seed are left. Refined oils have very little goodness in them.

However, they have a long shelf life and a high smoke point. This means they don't burn too easily or change chemical structure at high temperatures, which makes them suitable for frying at high temperatures. That's why they're so popular. But we are trying to move away from frying – especially at high temperatures! There is always a better way – think baking or grilling. If you want to fry, do it at a low heat and use just a bit of virgin olive oil. This will give you the same effect, with a fraction of the bad stuff.

Good fats

There are plenty of *really* healthy fats that fill us with energy and make our bodies thrive. I always try to get mine daily from a combination of **seeds**, **nuts**, **avocados**, **oily fish**, **coconut**, **eggs**, **grass-fed organic and wild lean meat**, **green veg** and **unrefined oils**.

Unrefined oils are usually cold-pressed (which means no high temperatures are used to extract the oil) and they are not chemically treated like refined oils. As a result, they might be cloudy, dark or strong in flavour. This is exactly what we want, because so much of the goodness of the base product – be it a seed or an olive – is still contained within the oil. They are loaded with antioxidants and vitamins.

Examples of unrefined, cold-pressed oils are **extra-virgin or virgin olive oil**, **hemp oil**, **flax-seed oil**, **walnut oil**, **pumpkin-seed oil**, **avocado oil** and **sesame oil**. Check the label to make sure it says cold-pressed, unrefined and preferably organic. All these taste great and will do you so much good! They are best kept in a cool dark place to prevent them going off.

Apart from avocado oil, which can be heated to high temperatures and is great for cooking, unrefined oils should

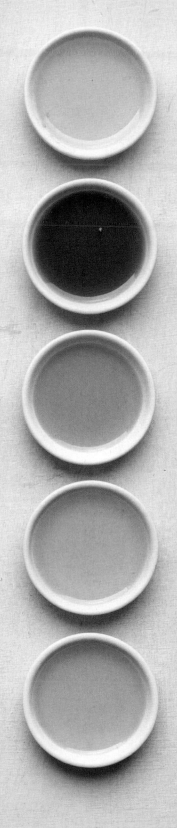

COCONUT: SURVIVAL FOOD

Coconut oil is so versatile, I always carry it in my survival kit. It has an antibacterial action, so you can put it on cuts and burns. You can apply it to dry, cracked heels and chapped lips. You can brush your teeth with it, to get rid of germs and bad breath. You can use it as a natural sunscreen if you have no alternative (it's around SPF10). You can moisturize your hair and skin with it. You can use it to oil your knives and other tools. You can use it as a fuel source to make a fire. And you can use it as a fuel source for yourself, when food is scarce.

Just bear in mind that coconut oil is rock hard below about 20°C, but becomes liquid above approximately 23°C. Room temperature is perfect. (Well, Shara's room temperature, that is!)

not be heated to high temperatures, or preferably not heated at all. They are best used in raw dishes, salads, raw baking, added to smoothies or for dipping crackers or vegetables in. You *can* cook with virgin olive oil, on a low to medium heat.

My all-time favourite oil, though, is **coconut oil**.

Coconut oil

The coconut is such an awesome survival food. Just the taste reminds me of all the times I've spent in the tropics (and the many times I've climbed coconut trees just to get at their life-saving fruit). The coconut contains an amazing nutrient-rich water that is full of rehydrating electrolytes and fluid-balancing minerals (such as sodium, magnesium, potassium and phosphorous). It packs a range of vitamins (such as vitamins C, E, B1, B5 and B6). Not to mention iron, selenium, a ton of fibre, a little protein – and lots of great fat. Coconut milk, cream and oil have become my main replacements for dairy products such as milk, cream and butter.

Coconut oil is mostly saturated fat. *But* it's one of the healthiest saturated fats you can have. It's easily metabolized, so it can be used as an immediate source of energy – great for people like myself who exercise a lot but are on a low-carb diet. It can also help raise your levels of HDL – the 'good' kind of cholesterol (see page 38). Instead of making you fat, it can help you to *burn* fat (if you don't eat too much of it). It can lower your chances of heart disease. It's an immune booster. It can support thyroid, prostate health and digestion.

Get the idea?

These are all reasons why I just love the stuff so much. If you really don't like the flavour or smell of coconut oil, there are several odourless brands on the market. But do make sure you get the proper stuff: organic, raw, virgin coconut oil.

Coconut oil isn't suitable for deep frying, but we want to avoid a lot of that anyway. It works great for quick stir-fries, curries, raw cakes, flapjacks and energy bars. It also works well in many oven dishes as it can be safely heated up to about 180°C.

Omega-3

Omega-3 oils are really important. They keep our brains healthy. They keep our moods high and help to fight off depression. They help keep inflammation in the body low. They keep our cells healthy and our skin flexible. They can reduce our risk of heart disease and cancer. They can help to lower bad cholesterol (see page 38) and decrease blood pressure.

Good sources of omega-3 oils are: **oily fish** (think **salmon**, **mackerel**, **trout**, **anchovies**, **halibut**, **sardines**, **tuna** and **herring**); **hemp seeds** and **hemp oil**; **flax seeds** and **flax oil**; **chia seeds**; **walnuts**; **pumpkin seeds** and **pumpkin seed oil**; **omega-3-fortified eggs** (from chickens fed a high omega-3 diet); dark green vegetables such as **spinach**, **kale**, **broccoli** and **sea vegetables**; herbs such as **basil** and **oregano**.

Oils that contain plenty of omega-3, such as flax or hemp, should be kept in the fridge. The oils are sensitive to light and heat, so protect them.

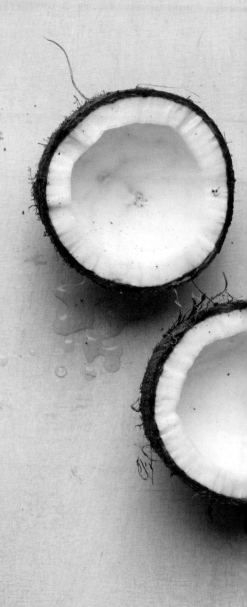

CHOLESTEROL

I never quite knew what cholesterol was until a blood test showed me I had 'above average' cholesterol levels. This was a shock – I wasn't smoking, drinking heavily or eating a lot of fried food. I exercised regularly and felt perfectly fit.

Like most people, I thought cholesterol was a bad thing. Was a heart attack lurking just around the corner? My quest for answers began.

What is cholesterol?

I'd always thought cholesterol was a dangerous, life-threatening substance. One of the real bad guys. But the opposite turns out to be true. Cholesterol doesn't just stop us falling apart, mentally and physically. Without it, we'd die. Fact.

Cholesterol is a fat-like, sticky substance that our liver produces. Our bodies also extract it from certain foods, such as eggs. Theoretically, the more cholesterol we absorb from our food, the less our liver makes. It is tightly kept in check.

Every cell in our body contains cholesterol (it is part of the membrane that holds the cell together). It's the building block of several important hormones, including the sex hormones testosterone and oestrogen (which give us our male and female features), and the stress hormones adrenaline and cortisol (which enable us to cope with stress). Cholesterol also plays a role in digestion. It's a part of 'bile' – a substance that helps us digest and absorb fat and fat-soluble vitamins (vitamins A, D, E and K). Without cholesterol we'd be unable to convert the sun's rays into vitamin D. It affects our mood by influencing serotonin – a neurotransmitter that helps us to feel happy. Oh, and it makes up 20–25 per cent of our brain.

What about 'good' and 'bad' cholesterol?

You may have heard about 'good' cholesterol (HDL) and 'bad' cholesterol (LDL). So what's that all about?

Cholesterol needs to be transported safely from the liver through our arteries to where it is used in the body. Imagine transporting butter. If you were just to put it in the back of a lorry, it would get stuck to the sides. If you put it in a plastic tub before loading it into the lorry, problem solved. You can think of LDL as being the tub that carries cholesterol to where it needs to be. HDL is the tub that carries excess cholesterol back to the liver, where it can be recycled or excreted via our gall bladder and bowels.

If more cholesterol is produced and carried around the body than is needed, and there are not enough tubs to carry the excess back to the liver, your blood result can show high LDL/low HDL. This *can* be dangerous – but it doesn't mean that cholesterol itself is a 'bad thing'.

So what makes high cholesterol levels dangerous?

The tubs of cholesterol are carried through our arteries. If we are healthy, the insides of our arteries are like a smooth tube, so the tubs can easily travel through. However, the insides of our arteries can be damaged by drinking, smoking, stress and unhealthy food. The body tries to repair this damage using repair material, which includes some of the cholesterol from the tubs. But the more it tries to repair, the more the smooth tube becomes bumpy and uneven. It's hard for all the tubs of cholesterol to travel through these bumpy, damaged arteries. They get stuck, and the bumps become even bigger. Over time, the whole artery can block up with repair material and sticky particles of cholesterol. If this happens near the heart or brain, it can stop blood and therefore oxygen flowing freely to these areas. Or, some of the repair material can dislodge and cause a blockage. All these factors can lead to a heart attack or stroke.

This gives us two important tasks:
- Make sure our arteries stay smooth and healthy, so if there *is* a little too much cholesterol, it can travel freely back to the liver and bowel for excretion.
- Make sure there isn't too much LDL in the first place.

How do I keep my arteries healthy?

Damage to arteries is mostly caused by 'free radicals' and 'foreign invaders'.

Free radicals are molecules that cause havoc all over the body, including in the arteries. They come from a lot of sources: fried food, sugar, fatty or processed meat, processed carbohydrates, cigarette smoke, alcohol, drugs, medicine, air pollution, stress, too much exercise, pesticides, unfiltered tap water, cleaning products, plastic packaging and toiletries, microwave use and burned food. Free radicals cause deterioration and inflammation, and are the starting points for disease in the body, including heart disease.

Foreign invaders are bacteria, viruses and food particles our bodies don't like. They can enter our body through a damaged digestive tract, lowered immunity or a poor diet and unhealthy lifestyle.

The good news is that free radicals and foreign invaders have an enemy: antioxidants. Antioxidants are like vacuum cleaners that suck up free radicals, repair damage, reduce inflammation and crank up our immunity so foreign invaders don't get a chance to sneak in. Antioxidants are found in almost all the healthy food discussed in this book and in the recipes on pages 111–230. We're talking: **fruit**, **vegetables**, **nuts**, **seeds**, **sprouts**, **herbs**, **spices**, **pulses**, **pseudo grains**, **raw dark chocolate**, **green and herbal teas**, **healthy unrefined oils and fats**, and **oily fish**. So by following the suggestions in this book, you're automatically taking care of your arteries and your heart.

How do I deal with raised levels of LDL?

An excess of LDL has almost exactly the same causes as damaged arteries. Everything on the free-radical list can prevent the liver from functioning properly. When that happens, it either starts producing too much LDL and not enough HDL, or it can't get rid of the excess LDL properly. Eating too much unhealthy fat and sugar can also make the liver produce too much LDL. So now you can kill two birds with one stone, because not only will eating the healthy foods in this book keep your arteries healthy, it'll keep your liver healthy too.

There are other things you can do to help. Excess cholesterol should end up in your bowel. Once it's there, it's either excreted (this is what we want) or reabsorbed into the body (this is what we don't want). This is where fibre comes in. Put simply, it binds itself to excess cholesterol to stop it being reabsorbed. That's why you may have heard that oats, which are full of fibre, help to lower cholesterol.

Other excellent sources of fibre are: fibrous vegetables such as **broccoli, cauliflower, kale, cabbage, peppers** and **onions**; fruits such as **apples, pears** and **semi-ripe bananas; nuts**; seeds, especially **flax seeds** and **chia seeds; beans, peas** and **lentils; quinoa** and **brown rice; psyllium husk** (a fibre available in health stores).

You'll find more information on fibre and how to look after your bowels properly on page 29.

What about eggs?

For many years we were advised not to eat eggs as they contain cholesterol. In fact, they're a good source of many of the nutrients that may help reduce damage to the arteries and heart disease, as well as supporting liver and brain function. They are a great breakfast food and far healthier than toast with jam or a sugary bowl of cereal with milk will ever be. Don't go eating omelettes or fried eggs every day, but in moderation they can be part of a healthy diet. Always opt for **organic, free-range eggs** – or, even better, **omega-3-enriched eggs**.

Statins and other cholesterol-lowering methods

You may have heard of drugs called statins which help to lower cholesterol levels. For many people – especially those with a genetic predisposition to high LDL levels – they can be useful, even essential. But they are not necessarily the cure-all they are sometimes presented as. They can have many harmful side effects, and do not fix the root problem of damaged arteries. I'm not saying that everyone on statins should immediately come off them – you shouldn't, unless your GP agrees. Just remember that if you have high cholesterol, your overall diet and lifestyle are very important factors in lowering it naturally.

You've probably seen spreads and drinks that claim to lower cholesterol. They contain substances called 'sterols' and 'stanols', which prevent the absorption of cholesterol from your gut. They may work to a degree, but I'm suspicious of all the gunk that goes into these highly processed foods. You can find the same sterols and stanols in natural foods such as **nuts, seeds, fruits** and **vegetables**. It's a far healthier way of getting them in your body.

Exercise

It goes without saying that exercise is healthy. See my book *Your Life – Train For It* on how to spend just 30 minutes a day getting all the exercise you need.

Exercise can lower cholesterol and help your heart. It increases production of HDL. It stimulates enzymes that help move cholesterol back to the liver. It increases circulation and strengthens the heart muscle. It increases immunity. And it reduces the fat content of the body. All in all, a very good thing.

However: you can do *too much* exercise, because even exercise creates free radicals in your body, and we know what they do. Always make sure you rest and recover before and after exercise (see Sports Nutrition, page 95 for instructions). This is crucial to keeping your organs and arteries fit. Don't run a half-marathon every day. Don't spend three hours a day every day pumping iron. If you do have several heavy sessions, take a day to recover from them.

Bottom line: exercise, preferably daily, but in moderation and allow for recovery time.

Conclusion

High LDL levels can be a sign that something in the body is out of balance and needs to be addressed. Cholesterol-lowering drugs or a cholesterol-free diet are not necessarily the answer, nor are cholesterol-lowering spreads and drinks. Concentrate on having a diet low in the bad guys and high in antioxidant-rich and anti-inflammatory-rich foods. And have regular – but not excessive – exercise. It really is that simple.

FLUIDS

If you want to know how important fluids are, try going without them. There have been a few times in my life when I've been stranded with limited water. The first of these was when I was in the military. We were in the desert, and our helicopter extraction was delayed by three days. We ran out of water completely, but we still had a 20km hike to our final extraction point. We were all delirious by the end. Dehydration can be agonizing and the need for water on the tongue becomes all-consuming. My sergeant could see that I, especially, was suffering. He gave me his last capful of water. That one act of kindness kept me moving. I have never forgotten his selflessness.

You can manage without food for just over three weeks (although I don't recommend that you try it!), but without water you're probably dead in three to four days. That's why, in a survival situation, the hunt for clean water should be top of your list. But this isn't just true in the wild. You can eat as healthily as you want. But if you're not drinking enough, or you're drinking bad-quality water, you're not headed for optimal health.

Why do we need water?

For all sorts of reason. Water carries nutrients and oxygen to our cells. It flushes out waste products. It regulates our body temperature. It lubricates various parts of our body – our bowels, for instance, to prevent constipation. It helps with our metabolism. It protects our organs and joints. It keeps our skin healthy and rehydrated. And it helps our brain to function. In short: water keeps us going.

How much water do we need?

There are all sorts of complex calculations you can do to tell you how much water to drink. On average, we need around 1.5–2 litres a day. But the truth is, how much you really need depends on many factors. How active are you? Have you exercised or sweated a lot? Are you in tropical heat or Arctic winds? Is your diet higher in meat or in vegetables (see my 'Water Rules' below)? Have you eaten

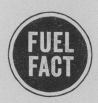

lots of salty or processed foods? Are you pregnant or breastfeeding? Are you ill, or do you take medication daily?

The bottom line is this: it's all in the colour of your pee! The best way to judge if you've drunk enough is to check the colour of your urine – it should be light straw coloured (although I prefer to think of it as the colour of champagne!). If it's darker, you need to drink more. If it's lighter, you're probably hydrated enough. It should also not smell very strong. If it does, it usually means it is quite concentrated. (Remember that intensely coloured foods like beetroot, as well as some medications or vitamin supplements, especially B vitamins, can make the colour of your urine darker or bright yellow, even if you are well hydrated.)

So, no complex calculations needed: just look down the loo!

The truth about tap water

In the wild, water can be both your friend and your enemy. You might come across water that looks incredibly clear and refreshing. But if it hasn't been properly purified, it can make you very ill indeed. Water's very good at hiding the bad guys: you often can't tell what it contains just by looking at it.

Tap water's no different. And while it won't poleaxe you, you need to know that a glass of tap water isn't quite what it seems. Chances are it's been recycled more than once. By which I mean that it may have already passed through someone else's body, then through a sewer. It might have gone through a factory, or been previously sold in a plastic bottle, then peed out and returned to your water supply. Now, I'm all for recycling water – it's a rare and precious commodity in many parts of the world – but in drinking recycled water we're drinking more than we bargained for. An average glass of UK tap water can contain around 300 chemicals. It should come with its own ingredients label. Although some of these contaminants are present in only small quantities, we drink a lot of water every day and it all adds up. All sorts of health issues, such as IBS or underactive thyroid, can be partially caused by the toxins in our water.

The solution

I aim to drink bottled water only. But be careful – a lot of bottled water brands are just filtered tap water. I go for artesian water, which means it comes from a mineral-rich underground source called an aquifer. It comes in top-quality recycled plastic or glass bottles. Chemicals from cheap plastic can leach into the water, so if you buy bottled, make sure you buy glass or good-quality recyclable plastic, which tend to be sturdier and thicker. And always opt for an ecological brand.

Quality artesian-aquifer bottled water is rich in all the positive minerals, like silica, which is great for your hair, skin and nails, and low in nitrates. This means it will be mega-pure and health-enhancing. Avoid the un-ecological brands or the bottled-water companies whose product is ground-water sourced – or even worse, just de-chlorinated tap water!

The best alternative to ecologically sound bottled water is a water filter. My favourite way of filtering water is using an activated-carbon filtering system or a reverse-osmosis system. You need to install these under your sink, but once it's done you only need to replace the filter every six months.

If you have a jug filter, make sure to change the filter regularly (you don't want the gunk to seep back into your water once the filter is full) and make sure to clean the jug every couple of weeks to prevent a build-up of potentially harmful bacteria!

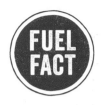

FUEL FACT

Here are some of the 'ingredients' found in your average glass of tap water:

Pesticides, such as nitrates

Drug residues, such as painkillers and hormones

Heavy metals, such as lead, mercury, copper and aluminium

Fluoride

Disinfectants, such as chlorine and trihalomethanes

Bacteria from your water pipes

KAY SAYS ...

I had a client from south London who had a very healthy diet but suffered from stomach pains with no clear medical cause. The first thing I asked her to do was to stop drinking water straight from the tap: I suggested she drank bottled or filtered water only. Within two weeks, her symptoms had almost completely disappeared.

BEAR'S WATER RULES

1. Don't drink large amounts of water with your main meals or while eating. Why? Because the food we eat is broken down by stomach acids and digestive enzymes. If we drink water while we eat, we dilute them. This means it takes much longer for our bodies to break the food down, and we may not absorb all the valuable nutrients within the foods properly. I drink water 30 minutes before (this also helps reduce your appetite) or an hour after my meals, then take a few small sips while I'm eating.

2. Thirst is often mistaken for hunger. If there is no reason for you to feel hungry (you've eaten a proper meal not long ago), drink a glass of water, give it 30 minutes, then see if you're still hungry.

3. If your diet is high in meat and low in fruit and vegetables, you generally need to drink more water. Fruit and veg already contain lots of water. Meat doesn't. It's also harder to digest and overloads your body with waste products – you'll need more water to help your kidneys flush out this waste.

4. Always check the colour of your urine.

5. Always drink filtered water, or bottled water from a reputable source.

6. Rehydrate before and immediately after exercising – you can lose more than a litre in fluids during a vigorous exercise session! See page 226 for my favourite rehydration drinks.

SALT

In ancient times, salt was a highly prized product. It was even used as currency – the word 'salary' is derived from it, as is the word 'salad'.

There is so much conflicting research out there about salt. On the one hand, you've probably heard that salt is 'bad' – that it can contribute to high blood pressure and heart disease. On the other hand, you may have heard that salt is absolutely necessary for keeping our bodies functioning properly.

So which is true? And should we really avoid salt at all costs?

Salt, in its natural, unrefined form, can actually be a fantastic health product. It contains over eighty elements and minerals that are essential to life, including iodine, magnesium, calcium, potassium and iron. However, salt in its refined, processed form – the white stuff commonly known as table salt – is not so great.

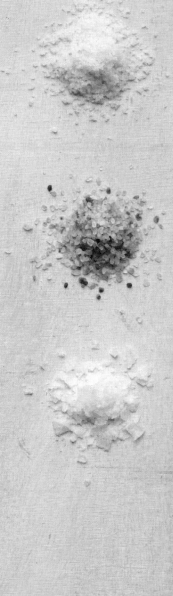

Table salt: what it really is

Table salt is the stuff we find on most supermarket shelves and in most processed foods. It is nothing more than sodium chloride – a chemically manufactured form of salt. The manufacturing process strips out all the precious minerals that salt contains in its natural state. These minerals are usually sold separately for use in other industries, such as agriculture or the pharmaceutical industry. That's one of the reasons unrefined salt is such a highly prized product.

After processing, other chemicals such as anti-caking agents may be added to table salt to keep it from clumping together and extend its shelf life. The product we're eventually left with has zero health benefits.

Table salt is not easy on the body and does so much more harm than good. It can disturb the fine balance of many body processes and of our body fluids, and it can contribute to health issues such as high blood pressure, heart disease, kidney problems, osteoporosis and impaired muscle and nerve function. Moreover, it is highly addictive.

WHY SALT IS GREAT FOR EXERCISE

I learned about the importance of using a good-quality unrefined salt when I started looking into how to rehydrate myself properly after intense training sessions. Unrefined salt is a great source of electrolytes – the ions that are present in all body fluids. The major electrolytes are sodium, potassium, chloride, calcium, magnesium, bicarbonate, phosphate and sulphate. They maintain water balance in the body and assist in nerve and muscle function.

When you sweat (or pee, or are ill with diarrhoea) you lose electrolytes. Unrefined salt provides most of what you need to replenish those that are lost after a good training session. So ditch the expensive sports drinks and just add a pinch of unrefined salt to your water or post-workout smoothie or shake for a cheap, natural electrolyte shot.

Unrefined salt

Unrefined salt is a complete package of wonderful minerals. For this reason, it can be very useful for our bodies. For example, the magnesium, potassium and calcium that it contains are known to have an anti-hypertensive effect. So, used in moderation, unrefined salt may actually help to *reduce* the risk of high blood pressure and heart disease, instead of increasing it, like table salt does. (When I say use in moderation, I mean: stick to the guidelines given in a recipe and don't use the salt shaker afterwards to add more. Always taste your food before putting any extra salt on it, and only do so if strictly necessary. Wean yourself off salt gradually and retrain your tastebuds to like the taste of the actual food, not the extra salt.)

Unrefined salt isn't usually sparkly white like table salt. Depending on the type, it comes in a variety of shades such as pink, grey, blue, red and even black. In fact, the whiter the salt, the less healthy and more processed it usually is. Examples of healthy, mineral-rich, colourful, unrefined salts are: pink Himalayan crystal salt, Celtic sea salt, Guérande or *fleur de sel* and Persian blue salt, or the healthier white varieties Maldon Sea Salt and Halen Môn. Most of these are available online, in health stores and even in some supermarkets.

Stay Below the Limit

It is recommended that we have no more than a teaspoon, or about 6g, of salt a day. This amount is easy to reach as salt is hidden in so many foods, both sweet and savoury – think breakfast cereals, breads, pastries, cheese, crisps, sodas, sauces, snacks, ready meals . . . Something as simple as a ham and cheese sandwich and a can of soda for lunch, combined with a ready meal for dinner, can easily bring you over your daily amount. Salt is also very addictive, so you should stop dowsing your meals in it before you've even tasted them. Start using fresh herbs and spices to flavour your food instead. If you use stock cubes, try to use those brands that at least contain sea salt.

Don't think that, just because unrefined salt has advantages, you can use as much of it as you like. Too much of any salt, good or bad, can be damaging (in a survival situation, drinking seawater can be life-threateningly dangerous). Everything in moderation.

GLUTEN & OTHER GRAINS

I find that bread is one of the most addictive foods on the planet. It beats chocolate by a mile. The smell of freshly baked bread is simply amazing – especially round a campfire after a hard day on the trail. On its own it doesn't really taste that extraordinary, but with something spread on top, it was a food I never thought I'd be able to drop.

In fact, anything made with white flour seemed to have that effect. Croissants, biscuits, muffins, doughnuts and pizza all left me wanting one thing: more!

Bread and other products made from wheat have been one of the toughest things for me to cut out of my diet. But, I have found that cutting out wheat and most products containing gluten has made a huge difference to me. Initially, though, I took a bit of a hit going cold turkey! I felt lethargic and the craving was intense. But after a while of falling on and off the wheat wagon, my body started to come alive! Suddenly I had way more energy, I was noticeably less pale, less bloated and more regular. It's cleared up a furry tongue, brain fog and helped me finally to lose most of my stubborn love handles (!), and it has been key to obtaining a lean torso and tighter abs. More than any other change I have made, dropping wheat has been the most beneficial for me, in terms of health, energy and looks.

It took me a lot of research before I was finally convinced to go against the grain (no pun intended!), but I've not looked back since. Of course, I have my cheat days – maybe once a week – and I love them. Sometimes a pizza or croissant hits the spot like nothing else, but I find I no longer crave wheat like I did before.

Bread and other white flour products contain several things that may harm you or your digestion: gluten, yeast, sugar and additives such as stabilizers, acids, raising agents, preservatives and emulsifiers.

What is the deal with gluten?

Lots of people seem to be gluten-sensitive or -intolerant these days. How come our grandparents were not gluten-intolerant to the same extent? Is this a modern, made-up symptom?

Gluten is a protein found in grains such as wheat, barley and rye. It is the substance that provides elasticity to dough, making bread rise and giving flour products such as bread, cakes, croissants and muffins their airy, fluffy consistency.

A gluten protein consists of two parts: gliadin and glutenin. It is gliadin that most people have issues with. In general, our bodies don't react well to it. This effect is strongest in those with coeliac disease, but even if you are not diagnosed with this condition, gliadin can do damage without you even realizing it. We don't seem to digest it well, and it has the potential to harm our intestinal lining.

Our immune system doesn't much like gliadin either. In some people, gliadin particles are capable of sneaking through the intestinal lining and entering the bloodstream. This can cause autoimmune reactions, inflammation, damage to other parts of the body such as the joints or the thyroid, and a whole range of other health issues.

With regard to the addictive effect bread seems to have, some research suggests that very small gluten particles can reach the brain and have a true drug-like effect. More work needs to be done on this, but there's no denying that bread is a highly addictive convenience food.

In small quantities, gluten may be perfectly OK for most people. However, in recent decades wheat, and therefore gluten, has become a much greater part of our staple daily diet – much more so than it ever was for our grandparents. We often consume it with breakfast, lunch, dinner and in snacks. We are told all the time that we need the carbohydrate energy. True – we *do* need carbohydrate energy, but not from such a nutritionally empty source!

Take a look at this example – an average food day for an average person:

- Weetabix or toast for breakfast (both contain gluten)
- 2 biscuits, or a croissant, or a muffin as a morning snack (all contain gluten)
- sandwich, wrap, bagel or baguette for lunch (all contain gluten)
- spaghetti, lasagne, a quiche or pizza for dinner (all contain gluten)
- a pint in the pub (usually contains gluten) or a granola bar after your evening workout (most contain gluten)

Because we are eating so many products containing gluten, the demand for the grains that contain it – especially wheat, but also barley, rye and spelt – has increased. And since we really like our products soft and fluffy, we want these grains to contain more gluten. So now, strains of wheat have been developed which, with the use of sufficient pesticides, deliver higher yields and have a higher gluten content. Great news for the supermarket shelves, but not so great for our bodies.

Modern wheat can contain around double the amount of gluten than wheat grown many years ago, but perhaps not even half the healthy vitamins and minerals originally found in wheat-grain kernels. This is why our grandparents may not have had all the health issues we have now. They ate better-quality grains with less gluten – and because the grains were natural, wholesome and filling, they invariably didn't eat as much and felt full sooner.

Hidden gluten

If you are diagnosed with gluten intolerance or coeliac disease and live a gluten-free lifestyle, you'll already know that wheat and gluten is hidden in loads of products besides bread. You will find it in many sauces, soups, processed meats, ready meals, salad dressings, sweets, crisps and beer, to name a few. The key is to scan the ingredients and look for 'wheat' or 'gluten' – it's usually highlighted in bold. (Or, even better, don't buy that kind of food!)

The recipes in this book contain no wheat and little to no gluten. The only exceptions are Marmite (sorry, I love the stuff, but I tend to have only a very small amount!), Worcestershire sauce (although there are gluten-free versions of this) and oats. Oats are *practically* gluten-free, and even some coeliacs have no issues with them. But to be on the safe side, if you are gluten-intolerant just buy gluten-free oats.

Gluten, however, is not the only reason I've given up wheat, bread and other flour products . . .

Sugar, salt and yeast

Most flour products contain sugar, yeast and salt. The sugar helps to activate the yeast, and the yeast helps the products to rise. Salt adds to the flavour. Both sugar and yeast can feed the bad bacteria in our gut and cause bloating and weight gain. Get the low-down on sugar on pages 29–32. And you can read on page 47 why refined salt is a no-no.

Additives

To lengthen the shelf life of bread and flour products, and to make them tastier and softer, a whole host of additives are often added. Some will be mentioned on the label. Others might not be.

It is not natural for bread to stay soft for more than a day, let alone a week! Travel to many other countries outside the UK and you'll find that unless you eat bread on the day it was baked, it usually goes stale and very hard. It's as unnatural to put these additives into our bread as it is to put them into our body. They can have a host of side effects. I recently checked the back of a packet of white flour wraps. Each wrap contained no fewer than fourteen ingredients – most of which were unpronounceable. And that is just in a simple wrap.

KAY SAYS . . .

Around 70 per cent of my clients appear to have an issue with wheat. Many are not diagnosed by their doctor, but when wheat is removed from the diet they experience vast improvements in their health. I had a client with severe ulcerative colitis, who tested negative for wheat or gluten intolerance. I still asked him to cut out wheat completely. He made an almost full recovery within three months, and lost several stone in weight.

Another client had severe reactions to the bread products she bought in the supermarket. However, when she travelled back to her home country and ate the bread products there, she hardly had any issues at all. It appeared that the quality of the wheat and the additives used to make the products in the UK were the real problem.

Gluten intolerance

Many people who are suddenly diagnosed as gluten- or wheat-intolerant may feel that their whole (food) world has crumbled. Going gluten-free means you can't eat anything at all, right? Make your way to any local supermarket and this misconception will be bolstered. The gluten-free section is always appallingly tiny and exceptionally expensive. It contains small breads packed in vacuum plastic which have the consistency of a rock, perhaps a single variety of chocolate cookie and some small bags of pasta that can cost up to three times more than 'ordinary' pasta. Expensive, boring and restrictive. And ironically, most of these have much more sugar in them to compensate.

So don't be fooled. Just because there's a 'gluten-free' section, it doesn't mean that everything in it is healthy or that the rest of your supermarket is loaded with gluten! The fruit and vegetable aisle, meat and fish, beans, pulses, rice, nuts and seeds and most of the Asian food section – they're almost entirely gluten-free.

So if you decide to go gluten-free, change your mindset. Realize that there are still more foods that you *can* eat than that you *can't* eat. And remember that going gluten-free forces you to steer away from unhealthy processed food and baked and breaded goods. There are some awesome wheat-free recipes at the end of this book to help stop those cravings, as well as some even better healthy alternatives to wheat-based bread and pasta, such as food made with buckwheat or almond flour (but more on that to follow...)

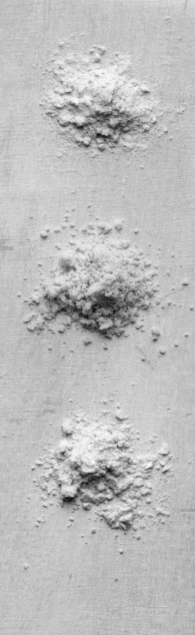

Bake your own bread

If giving up bread seems impossible to you, try baking your own. (Bread machines are reasonably priced these days and can do all the hard work for you.) Try using an organic flour such as **organic rye flour, kamut flour** (both are often better tolerated than wheat flour) or a good-quality organic gluten-free flour, such as: **buckwheat flour, rice flour, coconut flour, almond flour, chestnut flour, millet flour, hemp flour, quinoa flour, amaranth flour, sorghum flour, teff flour** or **gram flour**. Just remember that these flours don't rise like normal flour does and may require some experimenting.

Add healthy ingredients to your bread, such as seeds and nuts. You can also opt to make sourdough bread (or buy it from a decent baker). This is made with fermented dough. If prepared properly, the fermentation process will have lowered the total gluten content.

Beans, pulses, rice, corn and pseudo grains

After cutting out wheat, I started eliminating most other carbohydrate-rich grains and vegetables from my diet too, such as white rice, corn and potatoes, as well as beans and pulses. I then moved on to a very strict paleo diet for a while. This is a 'hunter-gatherer' diet, which avoids all grains, pulses and dairy in favour of mostly vegetables, fruit and natural proteins and fats. I found this really benefited my health and my waistline. But I also realized that having lots of bacon or low-quality meat, just for the sake of getting more meat into my paleo diet, wasn't actually particularly healthy.

Finding a balance between dropping the bad carbs and learning to cook with healthy replacements so that I can still eat 'normally' with my family has been the key for me. We still eat cakes and pasta and pizza, but now they are made with amazing, healthy ingredients. That's all. I was never going to win the battle of getting my kids to eat only vegetables, but a pizza made with a buckwheat base, or a pasta dish with courgette spaghetti? That could work! And it has. The family are all healthier and trimmer, and the kids have way fewer meltdowns now that the days of hyperactive sugar spikes are gone. (Well, almost gone – they tend to have a few moments of weakness, but I figure that's OK! It's all about inspiring those we love to eat better and more healthily by making the healthy food taste insanely delicious. If we do that properly, no one craves the crap!)

As a family we enjoy eating healthy pseudo grains such as quinoa, buckwheat and amaranth, especially on days when I'm eating vegetarian. These aren't really grains, but they do taste like it. They are wheat- and gluten-free (yes, even buckwheat, despite its name). They pack a punch of valuable nutrients. Each of them is a 'complete' protein, meaning it contains all the nine essential amino acids (see page 26). They are filling, satisfying and versatile, but don't leave you feeling bloated or sluggish. They're a great replacement in dishes where you'd usually use wheat or other grains. Quinoa has recently gained lots of popularity as a gluten-free pseudo grain, and I love it. But its lesser-known little brother amaranth also deserves a mention. It's similar in texture and flavour to quinoa, but smaller in size. It's not yet available in most mainstream supermarkets, but bought online it's often cheaper than quinoa. It's high in protein, fibre, iron and B6 – great for gluten-free porridge, or to add to soups, stews and salads.

I sometimes eat beans, lentils or chickpeas because they are quick, can be healthy in moderation and are a staple food in so many countries I travel to. I spend a lot of my time in South America, where it's hard to refuse their staple of beans and rice. Back home I use them sparingly, and I only occasionally eat organic brown basmati rice or wild rice as a small side to a dish such as a curry. For me, the fewer carbohydrates the better, which is why I tend to avoid white rice and corn. See page 29 for the low-down on carbs.

Although buying tinned beans and pulses may not be the healthiest option, it is by far the quickest. I don't eat a ton of them, so allow myself to use the odd can. But boiling beans and pulses yourself is obviously much healthier. Make sure to soak your beans *very* well (some for as long as 8–12 hours), drain them and rinse them. Then boil them in fresh water until they're tender, and drain and rinse once more. This makes them much easier to digest.

Soya

Although it might seem to be a good, complete source of protein if you're cutting down on meat, I don't eat a lot of soya. It can be hard to find soya products that taste good, and it has also been shown to be unhealthy in large quantities (so check your labels, because it's added to all sorts of food these days). Many soya products are made from GM crops, which I try to avoid where possible. I occasionally use organic tofu or tempeh in stir-fries on vegetarian days, or to make a quiche – see the awesome recipe on page 142 – and sometimes I use some soya in the form of a protein shake after a workout.

THINGS YOU CAN'T SEE IN YOUR GLASS OF MILK

IGF-1 – a growth hormone that causes the quick growth spurt in calves. This means it promotes cell division, so it can also stimulate the growth of cells we *don't* want to grow, such as cancer cells. Milk consumption may therefore be linked to an increased chance of certain cancers.

Antibiotics – most dairy cows are routinely given antibiotics as a preventative measure to stop them from getting ill. Residues of these antibiotics can end up in the milk. Not good news!

Oestrogen – modern farming techniques mean that cows produce milk continuously, even during pregnancy, when the oestrogen content of the milk is many times higher. There is a strong link between consumption of excess oestrogen and breast cancer.

MILK & DAIRY

We've been raised to think that milk is good for us, necessary for healthy bones, healthy teeth and to make us grow tall and strong.

I'm not so sure.

Around 70 per cent of the world's population doesn't digest lactose very well. But that doesn't mean milk is a great idea for the remaining 30 per cent. Humans only started drinking milk about 10,000 years ago. That might sound like a long time, but when you consider that we've been around for 200,000 years, you realize it's just the blink of an eye. We probably started using milk as a survival food in times of scarcity, but when there's plenty of food around, there seems little reason to rely on it.

Should we be drinking cow's milk?

Like all mammals, we drink breast milk when we're born. It's advised that human babies drink breast milk for up to six months to provide them with essential nutrients and help build their immune system. During these months our body produces an enzyme called lactase. Lactase helps to break down lactose, a sugar abundantly found in milk. As we grow older, we start to produce less and less lactase. Why? Because we no longer need breast milk to survive because we're now strong enough to get our nutrients from other foods, such as vegetables, fruit and meat. This is why you may start having issues digesting milk even later in life. Your body can gradually lose the ability to break down lactose properly. You can develop lactose intolerance or lactose maldigestion at any stage in your life – you don't have to be born with it.

Cows (and other mammals) are much like us. When calves are born, they suckle for seven to ten months. After this nursing period they eat grass to sustain them, and stop drinking milk altogether. Naturally, we should be doing the same. But we seem convinced that, after weaning, we need to continue drinking the milk of another animal to stay healthy. It seems a bit odd to me, and to many leading nutritionists it is becoming a clear danger area for health.

But isn't cows' milk full of nutrients?

Yes. It contains fat, sugar, protein and many important vitamins and minerals. However, most of the milk we drink is pasteurized, which means it's heat-treated to kill possibly harmful bacteria. This process also kills a lot of the valuable vitamins, enzymes and other beneficial bacteria present in raw milk. We then often take out most of the fat to make skimmed milk, which removes many fat-soluble vitamins such as vitamin D.

More to the point, though, milk contains lots of things that probably *shouldn't* be in our body.

Don't we need the calcium in milk for strong bones?

This is a bit of a myth. Strong bones require loads of nutrients, of which calcium is just one. One of the most important is magnesium, which is necessary for the absorption and metabolism of calcium. You can consume all the calcium you want – if there's no magnesium, it won't be absorbed properly. Milk is not the greatest source of magnesium. Vegetables – especially dark, leafy greens, as well as fruit, nuts and seeds – are a better and easier-to-absorb way of getting both calcium and magnesium into the body. So if you want strong bones, get some greens down you!

In several Asian countries, milk is not part of the staple diet. These countries often have much lower rates of osteoporosis than countries where milk is consumed.

Other health problems related to dairy consumption

If dairy gives you digestive issues, that doesn't necessarily mean you are lactose-intolerant. Lactose is the sugar found in milk, but it also contains two proteins called casein and whey. Many people have an adverse reaction to these substances. For them, drinking lactose-free milk is not always the solution. Cutting out dairy and dairy-related products is.

Recent research also tells us that the following health problems are possibly related to dairy consumption: asthma, acne, eczema, arthritis, breast cancer, prostate cancer, heart disease, diabetes and acid reflux.

Be warned: milk, lactose, casein and whey are added to many non-dairy items such as some crisps, processed meat,

THINGS YOU CAN'T SEE IN YOUR GLASS OF MILK

Sugar and fat – people love the taste of milk because 30 per cent of its calories come from sugar (in the form of lactose) and 50 per cent come from saturated fat. Excess consumption of sugar and fat are linked to obesity, stroke, arthritis and diabetes.

Casomorphins – these are proteins which, when broken down by the body, can have an opiate effect. They calm down the baby calf, but if you've ever wondered why cheese is so darn addictive, this may be your answer.

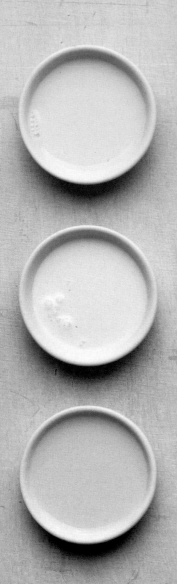

wine and dips. If you want to go dairy-free all the way, read your labels properly.

So what's the alternative?

There are loads: almond milk, other nut milks, coconut milk, hemp milk, oat milk or organic soya milk. They're widely available, so you could try a different one every week! They all taste a bit different – some work better in, say, smoothies or porridge, others are better in hot drinks. My personal favourites are coconut, oat and almond milk.

What about cheese?

If milk isn't any good, cheese isn't much better. A downer for me, because I love the taste . It has been difficult finding an alternative, but we've worked hard on creating some really great recipes that don't use cheese but still taste cheesy.

My favourite way of getting the flavour of cheese is by using a product called nutritional yeast flakes. Trust me: it tastes a lot nicer than it sounds. It's a de-activated kind of yeast, so it's fine for people with yeast allergies. And as well as the great flavour, it's full of B vitamins. It's available in most health shops or online, and it's not expensive. Just don't mistake it for yeast extract or brewer's yeast – they're totally different. You'll see that we use nutritional yeast flakes in a number of the recipes in this book.

What about chocolate?

The good type? Go for it. Chocolate made without the use of dairy and bad sugars or fats tastes much better than the regular kind. Check out the fantastic raw chocolate recipe on page 186 – you can buy the ingredients in most supermarkets and whip it up in 10 minutes.

MEAT & FISH

Many people think I must be a massive meat eater. I'm not. I choose pretty carefully how often I eat meat, and what type of meat I eat, for ethical as well as health reasons. Out in the wild I've found it hard surviving on plant food alone, especially when stuck in dry, arid land with little to no vegetation. Based on such experiences, one of my missions has been to show people how to survive when you have not much to eat besides wild animals. But when back home, the need for eating meat has become less and less.

Eating like animals

Although most people love to tuck into lots of different kinds of meat, I don't know of many who would eat meat daily (or at all!) if they had to kill or butcher the animals themselves. I know this from our TV series *The Island*, where those stranded often found it hard to hunt and kill their own food. But few of these people would have a problem eating a rasher of bacon or a pork pie back home. As a society, we have become very disconnected from where we find and source our 'meat'. Often we can't even tell what part of the animal the packaged meat we buy actually is.

We don't like to eat the less appealing parts of an animal – the brain, the tongue or the eyeballs. And we don't want it to look gross – rather as juicy, clean-cut and tender as possible.

Trust me: this is *not* how you eat meat in the wild, and it's *not* what your meat looks like before it's slaughtered.

You can learn a lot by observing how animals act in the wild. I've done this, and I've learned that if we were to eat meat like animals, we'd be eating *entirely* differently. When animals hunt in the wild, you'll usually see them going straight for those parts of their kill that we'd consider the least appetizing: think heart, liver, tongue, brain, eyeballs, bones and kidneys. The parts we think of as meat, they leave until last. This is because they instinctively know which parts of their kill are the densest sources of nutrients.

Don't worry: this book doesn't have a host of recipes using eyeballs or brains. (Check out my book *Extreme Food* if you're interested in that kind of thing!) I am well aware how difficult it is to move from a diet filled with bacon, sausages and chicken sandwiches to one dominated by cleaner, leaner sources of protein. My point is that if we want to eat naturally, we sometimes need to change how we look at things. Give the following some thought, and then make your choice.

Predator versus prey

While I am out in the wild, I consider myself prey as well as a predator. I could be killed by a deadly snake, catch malaria from a mosquito or be ripped to shreds and eaten by a grizzly bear or crocodile. But I also live off what Mother Nature has to offer, by eating the animals and insects that naturally come across my path.

That's how it is meant to be. We are part of the food chain. In nature there is a delicate balance. You hunt and are hunted. However, as humans we've evolved to such a degree that we hardly have any natural predators in our day-to-day living environment. But if we were put back out in the wild, it's unlikely many of us would survive easily.

So, even though hardly any animals eat us these days, we have taken animal-eating to an extreme. To satisfy our insatiable appetite for meat, we have developed very unnatural ways of breeding, keeping and killing animals. This far exceeds our nutritional needs. As someone who understands the importance of respecting nature and all the living creatures in it, and how we should keep the balance of the natural food chain, the mass, non-natural breeding and slaughtering of animals is something that makes me uncomfortable.

I'm not trying to convert people to a vegan lifestyle, although I actually do have a lot of respect for those who are vegan. But I do think that if we could all cut down our intake of meat, the world would be a much happier, healthier, cleaner and less aggressive place.

Meat to avoid

For the health of myself and my family, I now eat what I consider 'honest' meat. This means avoiding factory-farmed meat and processed meat.

Sometimes it's unpleasant to hear the truth about what's on our plate or in our sandwich. But I think people should know that:

- Factory farms keep animals in exceptionally inhumane conditions, under a lot of stress. If you think that eating the flesh from a stressed animal won't affect your own stress levels, think again.

- Factory-farmed meat comes from animals that are fed cheap, unnatural, pesticide-laden or genetically modified feed, which sometimes contains animal waste products (remember the BSE crisis?).

- Factory-farmed animals are often given a lot of medicines such as antibiotics, to keep them as disease-free as possible in the poor circumstances in which they live. The medicine doesn't just disappear from their bodies – it can end up on your plate.

- Animal agriculture is one of the biggest contributors to pollution, deforestation, water shortages and loss of biodiversity. Did you know it can take up to 10kg of grain and up to 20,000 litres of water to produce only 1kg of meat?

- Factory-farmed animals are bred to get as big and fat as quickly as possible. Many undignified methods are used for this. The end product isn't lean, healthy or honest.

I don't feed this stuff to my kids, and I don't generally eat it myself.

Processed meat is almost always made from factory-farmed meat, or the fatty leftovers thereof. It has a ton of additives, flavour enhancers and preservatives in it, not to mention a load of sugar, salt and bad fats that can seriously harm the body. So really try to avoid processed meat at all costs.

'Honest' meat

I love game. It tastes like it comes from the wild, and a lot of it does. Wild game chooses its own food from its own habitat. It is lean, clean, tasty, nutrient-dense and as organic as can be.

Some game, such as deer, buffalo or ostrich, is farm-reared. But even then it is mostly free from growth hormones, antibiotics and other medication and has usually lived under far better conditions.

Game has many nutritional benefits. Whereas farmed meats such as beef, pork or lamb have a much higher percentage of bad fats, which can contribute to inflammation and weight gain, game is much leaner, higher in omega-3 fats (see page 37), has fewer calories (if you're counting those) and has higher amounts of valuable nutrients such as iron.

Some people find game tastes quite strong. But please do try the two awesome venison recipes on pages 140 and 141. They aren't too gamey at all. The buffalo burger on page 148 tastes just like beef, only better and leaner. And if you get a chance to try ostrich or kangaroo, please go for it! They pretty much taste like a good lean steak.

Game can be a tad more expensive. But if the aim is to eat less meat, the meat you *do* buy can be of a better quality and a slightly higher price. (It doesn't *necessarily* have to be more expensive, though, especially when in season, when you can buy it in bulk and freeze it). Find a reputable butcher in your area, call ahead to place your order, then pick up your meat on a free weekend day and stock up for weeks ahead. This will save you so much time shopping around.

If game ain't your thing, always go for grass-fed, organic, free-range, naturally reared meat and poultry. Don't buy cheap chicken breasts. Instead, buy a whole organic free-range chicken from a reputable butcher. Eat the different parts throughout the week. This is proper value for money and the taste is so much better.

Be wary of rabbit. It might sound like a wild meat, but nowadays it is as intensively reared as chicken and other farmed animals, and under similar conditions. Make sure the label states 'wild' rabbit, otherwise don't buy it.

Fish

We're currently fishing the seas empty. Cod and chips used to be cheap as – well, chips. Now it's much more expensive because certain fish, like cod, have seriously declined in numbers. Or take the bluefin tuna, which can live up to forty years and weigh over 600kg, but which these days will rarely reach that age and weight since it has practically been fished to extinction.

But our appetite for fish has only increased, so fish farming is now a very big thing. Needless to say, fish farms use lots of unnatural methods to produce as much fish as possible in the least amount of space and time, and at the lowest cost. For that reason, farmed fish should be a no-no for you. Fish that have never seen the sea, a river or a lake and are fed on ground-up soya beans? No thanks.

However, I *love* to catch my own fish together with my boys, or share the catch of friends or neighbours. (Check out my books *Living Wild* and *Extreme Food* for the low-down on how to do this in the wild.) But back in 'normal' life, I only buy fish that is labelled as sustainable and wild. It will usually carry the MSC eco-label. Don't buy farmed or unlabelled fish unless you can ask the fishmonger if it's from a sustainable source. Please take this small effort – for the sake of your own health, as well as the planet's.

Meat-free

After reading a very interesting book called *The China Study*, I began to understand the importance of following a mainly plant-based diet to combat Western diseases and stay as fit and healthy as possible till old age. The book showed that we can get sufficient protein from a variety of plant foods. So it should come as no surprise that many top sportsmen and women, including body builders, choose to follow a purely plant-based diet (also known as a vegan diet). I know several of them and respect them highly. None of them looks malnourished, all of them are happy and healthy, they perform at the highest level and are ripped with muscles! I've incorporated a lot of their dietary habits into my regime, and I reap the benefits.

Whereas vegetarians choose not to eat meat but may still eat dairy, eggs or fish, those on a vegan diet consume no animal products, or by-products, at all. Animal by-products are hidden in many things these days, from alcoholic drinks to sweets, cosmetics, medicines and supplements. So you will need to read your labels carefully if you intend to follow a vegan diet.

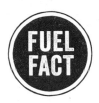

FUEL FACT

I try not to eat fish more than twice a week, because it can contain high levels of mercury, a heavy metal with very bad effects on your health. I tend to opt for smaller fish such as **sardines**, **salmon**, **anchovies**, **trout** and **mullet**, as these generally contain less mercury.

What to eat if you go meat-free

Going meat-free doesn't automatically mean you have a healthy diet. Crisps, chips, white bread, jam and sugary breakfast cereals are all animal-free, but not exactly healthy! Don't compensate for the lack of meat by eating lots of dairy, wheat, processed foods or sugar. This can have serious knock-on health effects. I have come across a lot of overweight vegetarians and even vegans!

If you're planning meat-free meals, make sure to eat a large variety of **vegetables**, **fruits**, **nuts**, **seeds**, healthy pseudo grains such as **quinoa**, **amaranth** and **buckwheat**, **millet**, **oats**, **gluten-free flours**, some **brown rice** and **pulses**, **avocado**, **sprouted seeds** and **beans**, **dairy-free milks**, **yoghurts** and **creams**, healthy **cold-pressed unfiltered oils**, **raw cacao**, **coconut**, **natural protein powders**, **organic tofu**, **green shakes**, **juices** and **smoothies**.

One advantage I have found of following a mainly plant-based diet is that I get to eat a lot more food without piling on the pounds. Some of my meals are massive, plates loaded with vegetables, giant salads and huge smoothies and shakes. I love to eat, so this certainly works for me.

We've got lots of awesome meat-free recipes in the recipe section. Some even taste meaty, like the Nut Roast on page 144. And there are millions of vegetarian and vegan cookbooks out there to give you further inspiration. So take the challenge and try to go entirely meat-free for the final week of my 8-week programme! I try to do this for a week every few months.

VEGETABLES & FRUIT

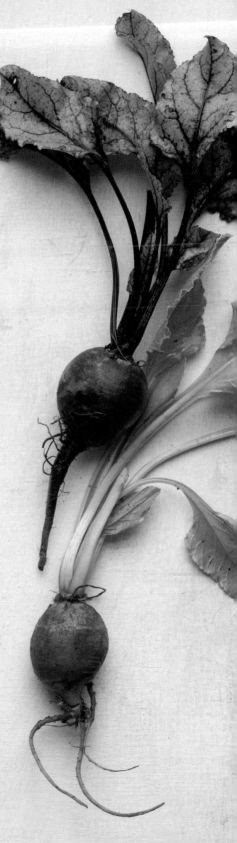

I grew up on vegetables that had been stewed for hours in our kitchen. By the time we got to eat them, they had invariably gone beyond limp and into mush (in other words, they'd been totally nuked!). The house smelt terrible once a day, and I learned to hate veggies!

I look back now and wince (and smile a little too!), but I also understand it was perhaps a cultural thing. And while I love my mum dearly, maybe I love her cooking a little less, even to this day! (Sorry, Mum! You're the best-hearted person I know – it's just that food to you was understandably about 'survival', not necessarily good health!)

It took me years, and a slow but complete re-education, mainly through books and positive experiences with like-minded friends, to learn that undoubtedly the best, most delicious foods I have ever tasted are natural wholefoods such as fruits and vegetables, beautifully crafted with the right flavours and spices to make recipes that explode in your mouth. It's the taste of good health and the wonder of nature.

But getting to this place has been an adventure!

What if I don't really like vegetables?

Trust me: I've been there. My first struggle was to make vegetables palatable. I did four things to help me achieve this: I started juicing them, I started making vegetable shakes, I starting eating them raw or only lightly steamed (not boiled to a pulp!), and I learned how to flavour the ones I disliked the most.

Juicing vegetables made me feel clean, made my skin clearer, helped my energy levels to soar and lessened certain aches and pains in my body. It ensured that I got a bucketload of nutrients in just one glass, and if I mixed in a little fruit juice I actually started to enjoy the taste of even the greenest-coloured juices!

I then went for the more adventurous route and added vegetables in their entirety to raw shakes. Broccoli, celery,

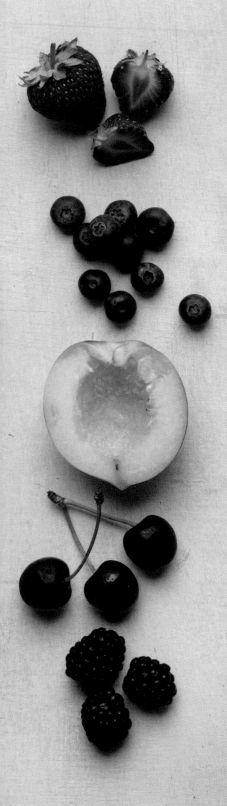

spinach, anything – always mixed with a bit of fresh fruit and water. This helped to increase my overall fibre intake and ease my digestion. I loved how, mixed with some lemon, apple and ginger, the shakes were green yet tasty. And they really filled me up.

Salads became my next big staple. I would chop in any raw veg I could find. So long as I chopped or grated it small enough, and mixed in some nuts, seeds, avocado or fish, I found I didn't mind the taste at all. I never much liked iceberg lettuce, but this was salad of a whole different genre (see my Rainbow Salad recipe on page 130). Salads even helped me to overcome my intense dislike of Brussels sprouts (see the recipe on page 125)!

I then learned how to flavour the cooked vegetables I'd never liked by using olive oil, balsamic vinegar, garlic, turmeric and other herbs and spices. Before I knew it, it was actually the taste of the vegetables themselves that became delicious. It is as if nature knows best! I'll admit that this process took a little time, but I hope the recipes in this book will help accelerate that process for you.

It's all in the colour

It goes without saying that vegetables have a gigantic load of health benefits. In my book, they should form the major part of any healthy diet. Our mums didn't force-feed them to us for nothing!

Plants contain a whole host of disease-fighting substances called phytochemicals. There are tens of thousands of these things, if not more. They often have complex names and they overlap somewhat with a term that may now be more familiar to you: antioxidants (see page 40). For ease of use and understanding, throughout the book I have used the term antioxidants to include phytochemicals.

Each different-coloured and -flavoured plant (be it a vegetable, fruit, herb, spice or pulse) contains its own range of antioxidants, with its own unique health benefits, ranging from heart health to digestive health and everything in between. Anything green is especially good, with many proven health benefits. As is anything 'smelly', such as cabbage or broccoli. But reds, yellows, oranges, purples, whites and non-smelly veg are equally important. The simple rule of thumb is: the more colours and the more variety, the better. Many antioxidants help us to ward off cancer, heart disease and other inflammatory conditions. They help me to keep my cholesterol in check. And they help to slow down the physical effects of ageing. Bonus!

So the moral is: don't stick to just one vegetable for your evening meal. Try to get as many different colours on your plate as possible. Stir-fries and rainbow salads are ideal for this. I try to eat 300–500g of vegetables every day – easy if you cut down on pasta and bread. Just fill up your plate with vegetables or salad, and unlike pasta and bread they will make you full but won't make you fat! Aim to have at least half your lunch or dinner plate filled with vegetables or salad.

Cooked versus raw

Unfortunately for my mum, cooking vegetables for long periods of time in copious amounts of water can really reduce the amounts of their disease-fighting substances. You end up pouring them out with the water, or they are simply boiled to death. Food-processing can do the same thing – think ready meals and vegetable soups in tins – so although tinned vegetables are still better than none, fresh or frozen will always be far, far superior.

There are a few exceptions. Cooking some vegetables for at least several minutes – carrots and kale, for example – may make it easier for the body to absorb their nutrients. But you should steam them, not boil them. (Juicing or blending can be a solution if you prefer to have them raw, as this helps break down the tough fibres and extract the packages of goodness.) Tomatoes may also be better heated, as this helps to release a phytochemical called lycopene, which is apparently great for your prostate as well as your heart.

Although I have considered going completely raw at times, it would mean a lot of work for me and for my family when I'm at home, because going raw involves a huge amount of vegetables, seeds, nuts and the like, never heated and mostly vegan. You have to eat a lot and it is quite hard work. So what matters to me most now is to make sure my kids and wife are happy to eat the vegetables I eat too, whether raw or cooked.

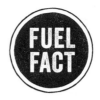

FUEL FACT

Mushrooms aren't really a vegetable: they're an edible fungus. But they do have enormous health benefits. They can help to boost immunity, offer many essential nutrients and are full of antioxidants. Grown or kept in sufficient sunlight, they can even be a natural source of vitamin D. Their meaty texture when cooked means they're a great addition to vegetarian meals, but I often slice them up raw in salads too.

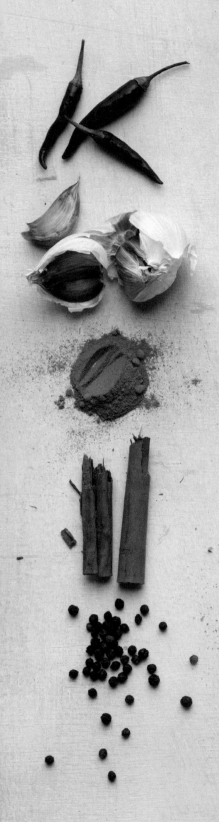

Fruit

Just like vegetables, fruits, with all their different colours, contain massive amounts of those health-promoting antioxidants. But they also contain fruit sugars. So, when juicing, it's better to use just a little fruit along with a lot of vegetables. When snacking on fruits, don't go overboard – dried fruit especially can be a concentrated source of sugar. I have two or three pieces of fruit a day – as seasonal, local and organic as possible – either mixed into a smoothie, juice or shake, or straight from the fruit bowl or tree.

Herbs and spices

Using herbs and spices really helped me learn to like vegetables. But not only do they add flavour, they also add a massive nutrient punch! Even that little pinch of turmeric or some chopped coriander can give you an extra shot of those important antioxdiants.

They have other great properties too. Many everyday herbs and spices, such as **black pepper**, **ginger**, **rosemary**, **cumin**, **turmeric**, **chilli**, **coriander**, **parsley**, **mint** and **cinnamon**, help with digestion, detoxification, circulation, heart health and much more.

So don't be put off by recipes using lots of different herbs and spices. Realize they contribute to good health and add brilliant natural flavouring. Just properly stock up your herb and spice cabinet and pantry. Job done.

Here's my definitive guide to all the health-giving herbs and spices you need.

Super-healthy flavour-makers: *always* **have these in your cupboard or fridge**
Black peppercorns, cinnamon, fresh chilli, fresh ginger, garlic, lemongrass, lemons/limes (or a bottle of lemon/lime juice), onions

My favourite herbs
Basil, coriander, mint, oregano, parsley, rosemary, thyme

And to fill up the rest of your spice rack . . .
Bay leaves, cardamom pods, cayenne pepper, chilli flakes, cloves, coriander seeds (or ground coriander), cumin seeds (or ground cumin), curry powder, fenugreek seeds, garam masala, ground ginger, marjoram, mustard seeds, nutmeg, paprika, turmeric

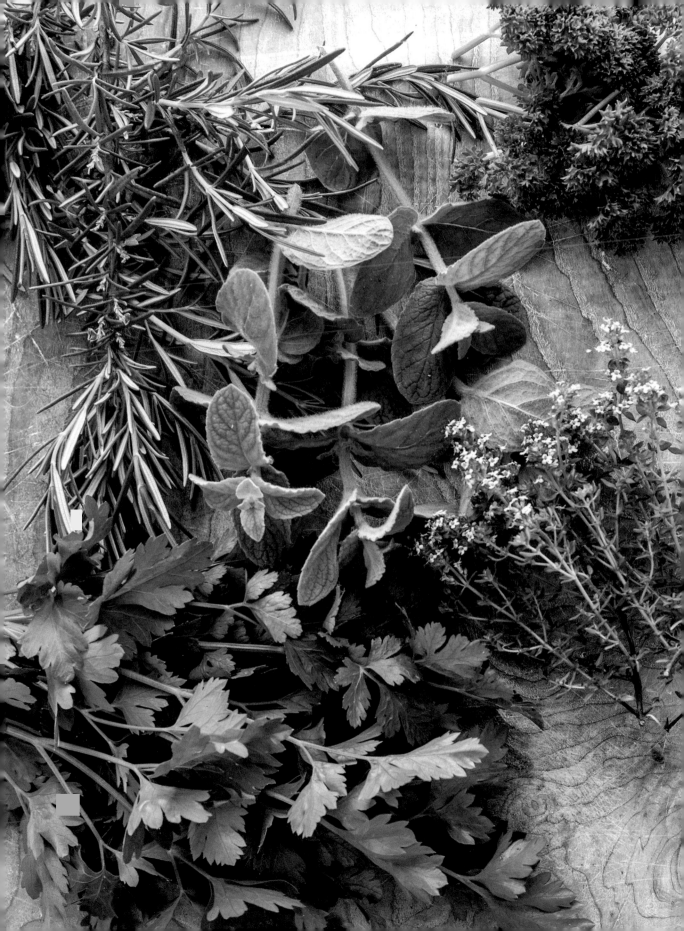

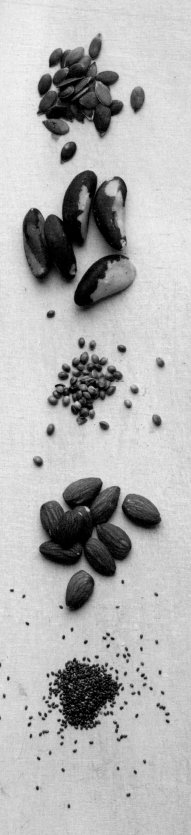

NUTS & SEEDS

When I was a kid, we used to eat nuts only at Christmas. We'd have a big bowl of walnuts and hazelnuts with the shells still on, and used a nutcracker to get the nuts out. And no one ate them much because no one could ever be bothered! Plus, of course, nuts were considered a very fattening food back then, so they just went hand in hand with all the other Christmas over-indulgence.

I've come a long way since then. Nuts and seeds are now part of my daily life. And coming across nuts when you're hungry in the wild is like stumbling upon buried treasure.

Yes, it *is* true that nuts and seeds are full of fat, but it's fat of the right kind. If you've read the chapter on fats (page 33), you'll understand that, instead of contributing to heart disease, these fats can actually help prevent it – especially when combined with all the other nutrients contained in nuts and seeds. They are an awesome health food. Of course, if you were to eat an entire bag of nuts or seeds on top of your usual diet, they'd be fattening. But eaten in moderation, as part of your daily diet, they do so much good.

Nuts and seeds contain many of the same nutrients as meat and fish. We're talking zinc, selenium and B vitamins, as well as protein and those important brain-boosting omega-3 fats. This makes them a perfect food for people who choose not to eat meat or fish.

Moreover, they are low in carbohydrates. If you've read the chapter on carbs (page 29), you'll understand why I think that's a good thing.

They are also full of antioxidants and other heart-healthy and cancer-fighting substances. Practically all nuts and seeds contain vitamin E, which can do wonders for your skin. They make filling, super-portable snacks – ideal for when you're on the trail or just rushing about in everyday life – and they don't mess with your blood-sugar or energy levels as they are a slow-digesting, satiating food.

You can eat these guys as they come as a snack, or use them in baking and cooking – I like them in smoothies, porridge and salads. You could spread some nut or seed butter on a rice cracker or oatcake, or have a spoonful straight from the jar with a few bites of banana (this can give you an awesome energy boost after exercise). You can use ground-up nuts or seeds as part of a gluten-free base for quiches or pizzas (see pages 142, 146). You can mix them into some home-made flapjacks or chocolate (see pages 174–5, 186) for extra nutrients. You can even soak and sprout seeds, which releases even more of the nutrients contained within them. Try this with chia seeds, for example.

My favourites

I like all nuts and seeds – they each have their own flavour and health benefits – but my particular favourites are:

Walnuts – they don't just look like brains, they're good for your brain too!

Almonds – a good source of calcium, so they're great if you're cutting out dairy. Almond butter, which is just ground-up almonds, is amazing on sprouted, flourless bread in the morning, with half a banana sliced on top.

Brazil nuts – the best plant source of selenium, which can help to fight off cancer and keep your thyroid functioning well. Just two or three Brazil nuts and you've had your daily selenium fix!

Pumpkin seeds – a great source of zinc, which is good for skin, immunity and especially the male reproductive system.

Coconut – this is actually a seed, not a nut. And it's my favourite one in the world! It's safe to say that on the TV show *The Island*, this is the food that contestants fall in love with the most, and which they crave afterwards back in normal life. Nature designed it that way – good for health, skin, heart, hair and morale! Read more about coconut on page 36.

Chia seed – an incredible discovery, and one of the few superfoods that really warrants the name. High in fibre, minerals, omega-3 and even vitamin C. A staple in my diet in smoothies, snacks, salads – you name it!

Sunflower seeds – great in flapjacks or, ground up, they can be used as a flour or made into a spread to replace peanut butter for those with peanut allergies.

Hemp seeds – they give you a complete protein and omega-3 fix. Again, think smoothies, salads and the like.

Flax seeds – another great source of omega-3, excellent

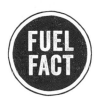

FUEL FACT

Peanuts aren't actually a nut, but a legume. They can cause a severe allergic reaction in some people. They may also contain a certain mould, invisible to the naked eye, which can be very bad for your health. They are often sprayed with pesticides too. On the upside, they are a really excellent source of protein, minerals, vitamins, good fibre and good fats. In moderation, they can be part of a healthy diet. My kids just love peanut butter, but I always choose the organic stuff with no added salt or sugar for them, and I am trying to wean them on to almond butter instead. (As an adult, I think almond butter genuinely tastes way better and more satisfying, and strangely I no longer much like peanut butter. Again, it's as if nature knows best and often guides us.)

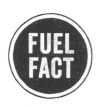

FUEL FACT

Some people find nuts hard to digest. It's best to soak them for several hours, or overnight, before eating. If, like me, you're a big nut eater, do what I do and keep a box of soaked nuts in your fridge, and change the water regularly.

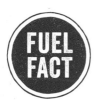

FUEL FACT

Salted, roasted nuts aren't healthy. But if you really don't want to give them up, mix a large bag of normal nuts with a small bag of salted nuts. You'll be surprised at how salty the mixture tastes, but you'll have helped yourself cut down your overall salt intake by a huge amount.

for your bowels, skin and hormone balance. You can use them ground up instead of eggs. (See the Flax Egg recipe on page 201).

Nut allergies

It's amazing how nut allergies seem to have massively increased in the past few decades. When I was young they were almost unheard of. Now it's reached the point where nuts are banned in most schools.

If you are one of the unfortunate people who has a nut allergy, it doesn't necessarily mean you are also allergic to seeds. This means you can still make many of the dishes in the back of the book, replacing nuts with seeds. If you *are* allergic to seeds as well, that is very uncommon and I recommend you see a nutritional therapist to check if something else is at play that may be causing your allergies.

Most people with nut allergies appear to be allergic to one or several particular proteins found in specific nuts. But not all nuts contain the same proteins. So it could well be that you can't touch cashews or pistachios, but that you are fine eating almonds or walnuts. Obviously you need to be very careful if you are at risk of developing anaphylactic shock, or your lips swelling to the size of bananas. But if your allergic reaction isn't too severe, I wouldn't immediately ditch all nuts after a single bad reaction. You could opt to do an allergy test to see which nuts and seeds are safe and which are not. This could enhance your culinary experience as well as your healthy-eating options. Just make sure you ask the advice of a healthcare practitioner if you plan to experiment.

Flax seeds, chia seeds, pumpkin seeds, hemp seeds and sunflower seeds are safe for most people. Start with those if you are unsure.

SUPERFOODS

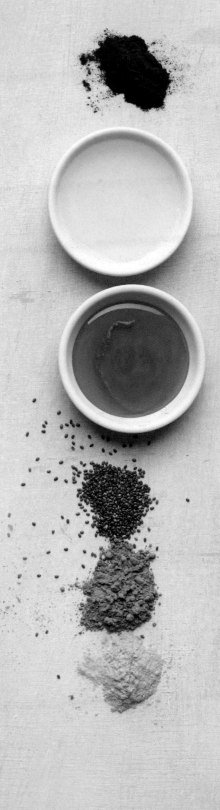

You've probably heard of 'superfoods' or 'miracle foods'. Some people claim that they can make us super-strong, reverse ageing, cure cancer and heart disease. Are these claims true? What is a 'superfood', anyway? And should we be including them in our daily diet?

What is a superfood?

There's no official definition of what a superfood is, and so there's no list of all the superfoods available. It's a marketing term, and like all marketing terms it can be misused. But *my* definition would be this: an exceptionally nutrient-dense food, very high in vitamins, minerals and antioxidants, which has health-boosting properties and provides exceptional health benefits. So, superfoods fight disease and keep you healthy and fit, which sounds pretty awesome to me.

Many natural foods we all know and love fall into this category. However, food companies and the media tend to hype up the exotic and unheard-of ones. These usually aren't readily available at your local supermarket. If they are, they tend to be very expensive and not necessarily worthwhile. Many food manufacturers add 'superfood' to their products simply to sell them – energy drinks with guarana, or breakfast bars with goji berries. But the truth is that having a sugar-loaded drink or snack bar with 2 per cent added guarana or goji berry isn't going to do you much good.

Despite the marketing hype, I think that using the word 'superfood' lets people know what kind of amazing foods there are out there in the world. Take maca powder: the Peruvians have been using this powerful, energizing root for centuries, but I hadn't heard of it until a few years ago. The world still has so many undiscovered treasures: berries from the jungle, roots from the mountains, algae from deep freshwater lakes, and herbs and mushrooms from ancient forests. As you probably know, I'm all for trying new things when they cross my path. If they pack an amazing health and energy punch, so much the better.

Health claims

Because many of the superfoods that get marketed are quite obscure, or come from faraway regions like the Amazon, not a lot of conclusive research is available regarding their precise health benefits. I'm of the opinion that if Mother Nature crafted something, and if indigenous peoples and ancient cultures have been using it for centuries, chances are it's going to do me some good. But I do bear this in mind: no one food alone is going to cure you of disease or work miracles, no matter what the marketing gimmicks say. Broccoli alone won't cure cancer, but adding it to your regular diet can certainly help you get and stay healthy. The same goes for the more exotic superfoods: they won't make you superhuman, but they can be a tasty, versatile, interesting and extremely healthy addition to your daily diet.

Too much of a good thing

Some of the most well-known, more exotic superfoods are **hemp seeds**, **chia seeds**, **maca powder**, algae such as **blue and green algae**, **spirulina** and **chlorella**, **mangosteen juice**, **baobab powder**, **moringa**, **ginseng**, **guarana**, **manuka honey**, **raw cacao powder**, **acai berries** and **aloe vera**.

I happily include all these foods in my diet. A lot of them come in powder or liquid form, or as seeds or berries, so you can easily test them out by adding them to a smoothie. These foods are best eaten as they come, not mixed in with processed food.

However, a little goes a long way. The key is not to have any of these foods in ridiculous amounts, and to vary them. Even the healthiest food can become unhealthy if taken in large quantities. Let's look at maca powder again. It's really tasty and gives you a great energy kick. But it also has the potential to influence your hormone levels, so you need to go easy on it – and you shouldn't have it late at night, unless you plan to exercise after midnight! Similarly, spirulina can have an effect on your thyroid – great if you have a sluggish thyroid, not so great if you have an overactive one.

You should also be careful if you're on certain medications, pregnant or breastfeeding. Some of these foods and powders can interfere, so if you're planning on adding something unusual to your diet, you should always speak to your doctor first, who may recommend consulting a nutritional therapist.

But the main thing to take home from this is that moderation is the key. Don't chomp down an entire bag of green powder. Simply add a teaspoon or two to a drink every now and again so you know it won't do any harm.

Let's not forget our readily available superfoods!
Superfoods don't need to be expensive or exotic. They are available right on your doorstep. Think **avocados**, **garlic**, **ginger**, **berries**, **cherries**, **oats**, **broccoli**, **kale**, **flax seeds**, **green tea** and **turmeric**. I'd consider all these to be superfoods: they are super-healthy, packed full of vitamins, minerals, antioxidants and many other goodies. Because we know them all so well, and they're not interesting enough for the media to hype up, we don't *think* of them as superfoods. But they're cheap, readily available, we know we can trust them and they're easy to incorporate into our regular diet. So these are the kinds of superfoods I tend to go for and which you'll find in the recipes in this book.

SUPPLEMENTS

In an ideal world, we should be able to get all our vitamins and minerals from whatever Mother Nature has to offer. But we're pretty far from living in an ideal world.

The stressful lives we lead can zap us dry of vitamins and minerals and have a negative effect on our digestion. The food we eat isn't quite what it used to be, since many crops are grown on depleted soil and most foods are now designed to taste better, not to have more nutritional value. They reckon that today we would have to eat eighteen oranges to get the same amount of goodness that we would have got from eating just one orange in 1930! The way fruit is picked so early, months before it reaches our fruit bowl, also conspires against us – especially when you consider that around 80 per cent of the goodness comes in the last 20 per cent of the ripening process (the vast majority of fruit is picked way before this phase nowadays).

In addition, we are exposed to more toxins and pollution, and we take more medication. This means more vitamins and minerals are needed to support our livers to allow our bodies to deal with these safely. We spend less time in the kitchen preparing fresh meals and rely more and more on pre-packaged food. Anything pre-packaged is bound to have fewer nutrients because it's so highly processed, or has been lying around on the shelf for ages.

To put it simply, modern farming and modern living are both battling against us, depleting our bodies of their much-needed vitamins and nutrients.

Here are some of the reasons you may want to consider taking supplements:

- you live a very stressful lifestyle
- you do a lot of air travel
- you rely on pre-packaged food
- you smoke or drink regularly
- you've been on several courses of antibiotics in recent years or take medication daily

- you feel run down and often suffer from colds, allergies or hay fever

- you live in a polluted city and rarely buy organic food

- you're in a certain phase of your life where you may need a top-up: for example, you may be pregnant, recovering from illness, going through the menopause or training for a marathon for the first time

I do a lot of air travel and have a very hectic schedule when I'm away. Sometimes I have little time to eat or sleep properly. This can take its toll on my body, my mind and my sleeping patterns. For this reason, I take certain supplements to make sure I have my nutritional bases covered at all times.

The safety of supplements

A magazine article about the amazing health benefits of zinc. A TV ad for the latest multivitamin. Your next-door neighbour telling you how wonderful he feels after taking high doses of iron or zinc. There are lots of reasons why you might run to the chemist to get your own supplement fix.

However, what works for one person doesn't necessarily work for another. It's not the case that *everybody* needs extra zinc or feels better on an iron supplement. And even though supplements *seem* harmless, it can be risky to self-medicate with them.

If you are on medication, real care must be taken with supplements, as some may interfere or interact with your medication. This can be dangerous. *Always* seek the advice of a doctor or qualified nutritional therapist prior to taking anything when you are on medication. The same applies when you are pregnant or breastfeeding.

How to know what to pick

Firstly, ask yourself what are you after, and why? Something to improve your overall wellbeing? Something for your immunity, digestion, skin or hair? Something to improve your mood, sleep, joint pains or bowel movements?

Once you know what you want, the best way forward is to go to a reputable health shop and ask for advice. Or speak to a qualified nutritional therapist, who will be able to tell you

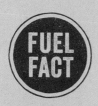

'The whole is more than the sum of its parts' *Aristotle*
Kale doesn't just contain calcium. It contains a whole range of nutrients that all work together *with* the calcium to keep you healthy.

Supplements are the same. Individual vitamins or minerals don't always work as well as those grouped together to work in synergy. So, unless specifically advised to do so by a professional, don't go for a high-dose zinc, a high-dose iron or a high-dose calcium tablet. Instead, go for a full-spectrum multivitamin, or a specifically designed combination of nutrients.

Most importantly, don't forget that unprocessed wholefoods themselves usually provide you with a nutrient package automatically . . .

precisely what is best for you. Try not to buy something yourself over the counter unless you have done some proper research.

Choose quality over quantity

If you think a £2 bottle of vitamins is going to make a world of difference to your health, think again. There are good reasons why some supplements are pricier than others. It isn't just a marketing con.

Firstly, vitamins, minerals and other nutrients come in all sorts of chemical forms. Some are very well absorbed by the body, some are not absorbed at all. For example, you can buy iron supplements in the following forms: iron fumerate, iron gluconate, iron sulphate, iron bisglycinate, iron citrate or chelated iron.

Confusing? You bet.

The point is that some of these forms are absorbed very well. Others aren't. They may even cause constipation or digestive issues.

So how to know what to pick? I'm afraid the better-absorbed forms are almost always the pricier ones. And if the ingredients or chemical form aren't specified on the label of your supplement bottle, it often means that a badly absorbed form is being used. Don't buy it.

Secondly, cheaper supplements can come in very compressed tablets which don't disintegrate very well, or at all. This means that a tablet you swallow in the morning could be coming out in your poo the next day. You'll be literally flushing your money down the toilet!

You should avoid supplements full of artificial sweeteners, flavourings or other additives. They can do more harm than good.

Quality really does come at a price when it's a case of putting vitamins in your body. Expert supplement companies spend a lot of time, research and money making tablets, capsules and liquids that are easy to break down and absorb. This is one of those occasions where it really pays to spend a little bit more.

What can I safely take without too much professional advice?

The following are generally safe for most people who aren't on medication, pregnant or lactating:

A quality multivitamin and mineral supplement – this touches all the minimum nutritional bases you require and can help in times of stress or when you're eating less healthily. Take them in the morning, as some vitamins can be quite energizing!

Probiotics – I don't mean the sugary, milky drinks from the supermarket. I mean a quality probiotic, either in powder or capsule form, from a health shop. These can aid digestive issues such as bloating, gas, constipation, IBS or yeast infections; they can help to strengthen your immunity and they can counterbalance the effects of antibiotics.

Omega-3 oils – especially if you don't eat oily fish often, it is really important to get sufficient omega-3 oils. They are necessary for healthy heart, brain, skin, nervous system and hormone function. They can help to keep your mood up too. Essential! Check the label for the total amount of DHA and EPA – these are the actual substances that do the health job. Look for about 500–1000mg per day combined of DHA and EPA. There are vegan versions available too if fish oil doesn't float your boat.

Milk thistle – this herb protects the liver and can help it to deal with all the toxins we are exposed to on a daily basis as proven by plentiful research. Or if you have a party weekend coming up, it can help ease that hangover a bit more quickly!

Turmeric – this is one of the healthiest roots on the planet and a great flavour-maker in curries. But if curries aren't your thing, you can also buy it in capsule form. Turmeric is good for immunity and for inflammation; it's super-high in antioxidants, is great for the brain, heart, joints and much more. An all-round health bomb. It is best taken in combination with black pepper to aid absorption.

Vitamin D – I am fortunate enough to travel a lot and get a decent fix of sunshine regularly, which is a great source of vitamin D. However, many people don't get proper exposure to regular sunlight. Food rarely provides us with sufficient amounts of this vitamin so, especially in the darker months from October to April, it's a good idea to get a daily top-up of a good-quality vitamin D. You could also take it in the summer months if you don't get to go out much, or if you wear a heavy sunblock at all times (which can prevent the absorption of vitamin D from the sun).

Vitamin C – unlike most animals in the wild, humans are not capable of producing vitamin C in their body. And as we are eating less and less fresh food, a top-up, especially in the winter months, can be a great idea to help boost overall immunity and to ward off any colds and flus.

Herbs

In the wild, I've used lots of herbs and plants for medicinal reasons (check out my books *Living Wild* and *Born Survivor* for more on that). But this isn't just useful knowledge when you're miles from civilization.

Did you know that most medicines prescribed by doctors are synthesized copies of one or more chemical components originally found in a herb or plant? Mother Nature is a full medicine cabinet! Herbs can be incredibly potent. I find that they can be superior to some supplements. Many health shops sell herbs in tinctures or capsules. Get some professional advice on which herbs to choose for your specific condition and be prepared to be amazed by the outcome.

No excuses

There are so many more supplements, powders, tinctures and herbs that could possibly combat some physical symptoms you might be dealing with. And I highly recommend you do some research or ask a professional in the field what could be good for you.

However, a very important message to take home from this chapter is: *do not use supplements as an excuse not to eat healthily*.

Supplements can be used in addition to your daily diet, as a means to alleviate certain ailments when recommended by a professional, or as a top-up in times of need. But they should never be used as a replacement for eating healthy foods. The best supplement truly is eating clean, lean, organic wholefoods as found in nature!

STIMULANTS

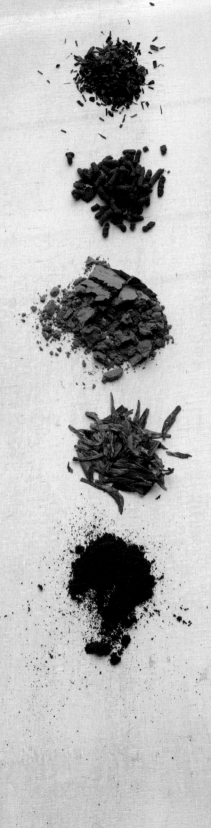

Addictive and stimulating substances such as chocolate, coffee and alcohol have become an integral part of our society. Our brains are programmed to love them – and also to get hooked on them. It seems to be part of our coping mechanism for life. And I include myself in this category for sure! These substances can give us instant pleasure, they can lessen pain, make us more sociable and help us push on in times of stress. No wonder people – some more than others – find them hard habits to kick.

But the simple truth is that too much too often can also damage our health and stop our brain working properly. These substances can interfere with rational thinking, enhance our stress levels, make us gain weight and put a strain on our body. So, the temporary bliss and stimulating effects don't last for ever, and they do leave their scars. That's why I have worked hard in my attempt to reduce my dependence on them.

So how do I deal with chocolate, coffee and alcohol? Do I avoid them completely? Put them all in the 'bad-for-me' category? Absolutely not. I'm not out to punish myself. I just keep in mind that moderation and purity are key.

Chocolate

I've always loved chocolate, and I consider it to be an amazing health food. You just have to pick your chocolate carefully.

The most unhealthy part of eating an average chocolate product is not the chocolate itself, but the other ingredients in it. We're talking white sugar, cream or milk, and a lot of fat – not to mention that the cacao bean itself has probably been heavily processed. Chocolate contains several substances – for example, theobromine, tryptophan and phenylethylamine – that can have a happy, relaxing, comforting or stimulating effect on the brain and our mood. It also contains magnesium, a mineral of which some women may need more once a month, which could explain those PMS chocolate cravings. However, many chocolate cravings are probably caused by the two other super-addictive substances in an average chocolate bar: white sugar and dairy. Both are bad, and mega-fattening. But don't panic! Help is at hand.

Chocolate in its organic, raw, unprocessed form, however – often referred to as raw cacao – is super-rich in antioxidants and minerals, can be exceptionally healthy and, if used correctly, is just so delicious! There's evidence that consuming a small amount of raw cacao on a daily basis can be extremely beneficial to heart health and can help lower blood pressure.

So, rather than trying to abstain from chocolate for a week before having a big binge of 'bad' chocolate, have a little of the right kind every day. Raw cacao is the way forward. It's available online and in most health shops. You want the organic, unsweetened stuff, and it's what we use in all the amazing chocolate recipes in this book. (The Chocolate Brownies on page 188 can be prepared in minutes and I hope they'll convince you never to buy a processed chocolate bar again.) And if you're a real dark chocolate fan, try snacking on some cacao nibs. These are cacao beans smashed up into little pieces. They give you an amazing chocolate kick without the added sugar rush. Great to bring with you when you are out and about or travelling, or even for a mid-morning pick-me-up. My favourite, though, is without doubt the plain old chocolate squares made from raw cacao, maple syrup and coconut oil poured into an ice-cube tray on page 186.

Coffee

Coffee has many similarities to chocolate: in its pure, organic form (we're talking freshly ground organic coffee beans) it can have many health-promoting properties. It contains small amounts of important nutrients like B vitamins, magnesium and a whole host of disease-fighting antioxidants. It can have a positive effect on your brain and body, helping with both mental and physical performance.

As with chocolate, it is often the extra ingredients in a cup of coffee that you have to look out for. Lattes and cappuccinos full of milk, iced coffees with cream and sugar, speciality coffees with flavoured syrup shots or whipped cream on top: damaging and fattening.

However, coffee itself, even drunk black with no sugar,

can have negative side effects. It can contribute to anxiety, insomnia, dehydration, heartburn and even weight gain. Coffee contains caffeine, which is a powerful stimulant. Caffeine can stimulate our bodies to produce adrenaline. Adrenaline is our fight-or-flight hormone. It stems from primal days when we still had to run away from tigers or fight off other threats. Not only does adrenaline raise our heartbeat and blood pressure, prepping us for action, it also causes a release of glucose into the bloodstream. This glucose can be used as instant energy by our muscles – great if you *really* need to run away from a tiger or fight off a predator, but if you don't, the unused glucose is later stored as fat. Yes, that caffeine *can* make you fat! The worst time to drink coffee is when you are sitting at your desk. Instead, drink it right before a vigorous exercise session when it can help with endurance and performance. Coffee is often used as a mental stimulant, but don't rely on this: caffeine is addictive, and you'll only need more and more of it to maintain the same effect. A balanced body should cause a balanced mind.

Coffee is harsh on the stomach and digestive system and can contribute to indigestion and acid reflux. If you have such digestive issues, stick to no more than one cup a day. And if you're naturally anxious or suffer from insomnia, coffee may not be for you. Most decaffeinated coffee has gone through an extensive chemical process to have the caffeine extracted. Not a healthy option. It's still mildly stimulating, though, and still very harsh on the stomach. If you're looking for a mental boost, go for green tea instead.

To give your energy levels, blood sugar and digestive system a break, we're cutting coffee down to a minimum in my 8-week eating plan (see page 233). If you drink a lot of coffee, you may initially get some headaches, but these are just short-lived withdrawal symptoms showing you how addicted you really were. You'll be amazed at how much more energized you'll feel once you've cut it down. I know this from experience – the first week was hell, but now the occasional coffee is a treat, not a compulsory daily fix, and it makes it way more pleasurable like that, I promise.

There are many coffee substitutes these days, some with amazing health benefits, some with fantastic tastes, some with both or neither. If you feel you have a coffee addiction,

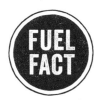

Neither coffee nor alcohol contributes to your daily recommended fluid intake. They both dehydrate the body – you'll notice this in the colour and smell of your pee. If you drink coffee or alcohol, you should always drink more water too, in order to compensate.

try one of my favourites: **chicory coffee**, **dandelion root coffee**, **Mediterranean herbal coffee**, any herbal teas and loose-leaf **green tea** or **white tea**. You could also try the following, which are super-energizing but not caffeine-free: **hot maca powder**, **matcha green tea**, **guayusa** and **yerba mate**. Shara's favourite is **red bush tea** or **rooibos** – and she looks smoking hot on it!

Alcohol

As a student I definitely went through a phase of hanging out, eating crappy food, drinking quite a bit of alcohol and smoking cigarettes more than is ever smart. This changed when I made the decision to put myself up for 21 SAS training. Simply put, maintaining that unhealthy student lifestyle was not going to be possible if I wanted to join the elite. That decision, and the health changes I went through subsequently, changed my entire outlook on alcohol, cigarettes and the effect they have on our health, fitness, longevity and happiness.

Alcohol helps us lose our inhibitions and, if I am honest, as a young man I did sometimes feel a bit of an outsider. I didn't want to be like everyone else, but I didn't know what that really meant. When I went out socially, I would use alcohol to give me the courage to walk my own path. But over time, and through developing solid foundations in my life through my Christian faith, I have found a quiet confidence in individuality and I no longer have to rely on alcohol.

Alcohol is highly addictive. Excess consumption can kill brain cells, cause severe dehydration, contribute to acid reflux, stomach ulcers, sleep disturbances, inflammation, diabetes, high cholesterol and heart disease. It also steals essential vitamins and minerals from our body.

But one of the biggest problems with alcohol is the effect it has on our liver. And our liver never complains. If we've had a few too many, we may feel it in our head, our stomach or even our legs, but our liver doesn't physically hurt when we've drunk too much, even though it is the organ most affected. This is a pertinent point to note; I'm sure that if we were to experience severe liver pain each time we over-indulged, we'd be far less likely to do it.

What's more, alcohol is full of sugar, or is converted into sugar very quickly by our bodies. I know people who claim not to have a sweet tooth, yet they drink alcohol almost every night of the week. It's their hidden sugar fix.

The blood-sugar imbalances that alcohol causes, paired with loosened inhibitions, have another side effect: breaking our determination not to eat unhealthy things. When was the last time you tucked into a salad after a night in the pub? You're much more likely to eat fatty, deep-fried, salty foods after you've been drinking alcohol. Or to raid the fridge late at night (I'm guilty of this too!).

There is some research that claims two glasses of alcohol a day may lower the risk of heart disease and other illnesses, but I wouldn't ever bank your health on this. What I do know is that if you are overweight, smoke and rarely exercise, two glasses of red wine a day probably won't save you from an impending heart attack.

You don't have to be teetotal. I'm not. But as with everything else, you just have to use your common sense. Buy good-quality alcohol, like organic red wine or a local organic beer or cider. Cherish it and save it for cheat days or special occasions only.

If you drink alcohol daily, the 8-week eating plan (see page 233) will help you cut down. Give your liver a break, then don't pick up where you left off. Form new and better habits. It won't be easy at first, but worthwhile journeys often have a little short-term pain at the start. Making alcohol or strong coffee a treat rather than a daily – and little-appreciated – habit will make a huge difference to your overall health.

ORGANIC FOOD

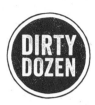

These are the fruits and vegetables that are most heavily sprayed. You may expose yourself to more than sixty harmful chemicals by eating these, so it's much better to buy the organic version:

apples
berries and cherries
carrots
celery
grapes
kale
lettuce and cucumber
nectarines and peaches
pears
peppers
potatoes
spinach

The availability of all sorts of food has massively increased these days. We can get our hands on almost anything. Most seasonal vegetables and fruits are available all year round and practically any other food we like can be imported from abroad. But there's a flip side to this abundance: the quality of most of the food we buy is not quite the same as it used to be.

We want perfect

You might not immediately notice this quality drop when shopping at your local supermarket. The fruit and vegetables all look beautiful and shiny. They are all the same shape, colour and size. But this is not what real food looks like in nature. Just ask someone who grows their own vegetables, or visit an organic farmers' market and you'll see it's true.

We tend to shop with our eyes, not our brains. Even amid this perfection, we'll still hunt for the biggest bananas, the shiniest apples and the straightest cucumbers. And that's why supermarkets won't stock less-than-perfect-looking food, even if the imperfect-looking stuff is perfectly edible. It's crazy.

But looks can be deceptive. Have you ever wondered how it is possible for all your apples or cucumbers to be exactly the same shape, colour and size? You probably won't be surprised to learn that something more sinister is going on.

We want sweet

It's not just the size and shape of our fruit and veg that don't seem good enough. There has also been an increasing consumer demand for sweeter-tasting, less tart or bitter varieties of fruits and vegetables, preferably with no pips: think grapes. New growing techniques, fertilizers, pesticides and all sorts of other interesting methods are used to create the tastes we want. However, it is often the bitter or tart substances in fruits and vegetables that are exceptionally good for our health and that can help to combat disease.

So, we're creating more unnaturally produced, chemical-laden food with better – or at least sweeter – tastes but fewer nutrients and health-protecting properties.

We want more

Not only do we want our food to look perfect and taste sweeter, there are also so many more mouths to feed these days. Food needs to be mass-produced in the most cost-effective way. But this comes at a price. Again, producers use a variety of new growing techniques, chemical fertilizers and pesticides. Fruit is picked before it is ripe, or we import it from countries whose pesticide laws may not be as strict as ours, and sometimes we store it for months. Crops may be grown in soil that is almost devoid of nutrients.

All this is at the expense of the quality of our food, no matter how good it looks. Did you know that an average peach fifty years ago could contain about fifty times more vitamin C than an average peach today? Today's peach is bigger, shinier and sweeter, but it's far less nutritious.

Pesticides

Pesticides can do crazy things to the body. In minute amounts they are legal and won't kill you. In large amounts, they certainly would. Over time, pesticides tend to accumulate in the body and can do a whole lot of damage, slowly but surely. They can contribute to a range of illnesses, from Parkinson's, thyroid conditions and hormone imbalances to cancer. The toxins can also make you fat. Not only do they meddle with your metabolism and hunger hormones, if you ingest more toxins than your body can handle it stores the excess toxins away in fat cells. If there isn't enough storage space, your body will simply create more fat. That's why eating food loaded with pesticides can lead to weight gain.

I convinced myself to eat more organically by giving the foods I bought different labels in my head. Instead of thinking of it as 'conventionally grown food', I started labelling it as 'food with added pesticides'. When you start thinking like that, it becomes a no-brainer.

The Dirty Dozen and Clean Fifteen

Some fruits and vegetables are more heavily sprayed than others. So if you can't go organic all the way, make a note of the lists on these pages and stick them in your wallet to help you when you go shopping. (Remember that if your local farm does not carry the official organic label, they may simply be in the process of trying to acquire it. It's always worth asking if

CLEAN 15

These are the fruits and vegetables least affected by pesticides. You could get away with buying these non-organic:
asparagus
aubergines
avocados
broccoli
cabbages
grapefruits and lemons
kiwis
mangoes
melons
mushrooms
onions and garlic
peas
pineapples
sweet potatoes
tomatoes

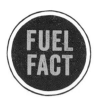

Genetically modified food

There does not seem to be conclusive research showing that genetically modified food is safe in the long run. It's still banned in many countries worldwide. It worries me that GM crops may endanger insect species, especially bees. And if you think GM crops need fewer pesticides, think again. Super-weeds and super-bugs are now popping up that are resistant to GM crops. This means even more potent pesticides are needed to ward them off.

My opinion is that you shouldn't meddle with Mother Nature – she usually knows best. Check your labels, and opt for no GM exclusively.

they adhere to organic standards despite the lack of a label.)

Bananas used to be in the Clean 15 because of their thick skin. But now they are so heavily sprayed that the soil they grow in is highly contaminated and the toxins tend to get absorbed into the banana flesh as they grow. Also, many companies use a fast-ripening technology where bananas may be sprayed or even injected with chemicals to help them ripen. Nice.

But it's not all bad!

Thankfully, however, there are many farmers who still believe in natural farming methods and don't worry about growing odd-shaped or odd-sized vegetables and who look after the soil, making sure to rotate crops to maintain optimal mineral levels in the ground. Farmers who care for the environment, for animal welfare and for our health by using few pesticides or other harmful substances. It's called organic farming.

There doesn't seem to be sufficient evidence to show that organically grown foods contain more vitamins and minerals than conventionally grown ones. But that doesn't mean they aren't healthier. An organically grown apple may contain the same amount of vitamin C as a conventionally grown one, but it contains far fewer harmful chemicals. The more harmful chemicals you ingest, the more vitamins you need to help your body get rid of them. Catch 22.

But isn't eating organic more expensive?

Farming is a tough business. But it's an even tougher, more tightly regulated and far lengthier process for farmers to get an organic stamp on their produce. So yes, organic produce comes at a price.

But *not* eating organic comes at a price, too. Pesticides are invisible to the eye, but not to your body. Not to mention the detrimental effects they have on nature. Is your health and that of your family and your environment important enough to invest a little more in better-quality food?

And in any case, it's beyond question that if you ditch expensive, processed food, ready meals and dodgy snacks in favour of the healthy, energy-giving fuel in this book, your health and that of your family will significantly improve. If organic food appears expensive, think of it in these terms and suddenly it won't seem like such an extravagance after all.

MICROWAVES

I've heard all sorts of rumours about microwave ovens – the
Nazis invented them, the Russians banned them, people
with pacemakers shouldn't go near them. It's hard to
separate the fact from the fiction. For me, the big questions
are whether they're safe to cook your food, and whether
'microwave meals' are good, energy-boosting fuel.

How microwaves work

I hardly ever use a microwave these days, and looking at
how they work is very revealing. They radiate very short
waves of electromagnetic energy which travel at the speed
of light and penetrate your food. This causes the molecules
in your food – and especially the water molecules – to
vibrate. These vibrations create heat. The longer you leave
your microwave on, the faster the vibrations and the more
heat generated. This eventually warms, or even cooks,
your food.

Ingenious. But also scary. Because microwaves are a
form of radiation. And the word 'radiation' never sits that
well with me.

Radiation is everywhere. We can't see it, but it's there,
and many forms have been proved to be bad for our health
and we know it can do harm when we are constantly
exposed to it. For that reason, just as we shouldn't have too
many X-rays or spend too long soaking up the ultra-violet
radiation of the sun, so we should avoid over-using our
microwave ovens.

The other question is, does microwaving our food
reduce its nutrient content? So far as I can tell, the science
is inconclusive on this one. But I still try to avoid them.
The radiation argument alone won me over!

Do microwaves really save time?

Yes. Marginally. But I mean, marginally. Because by the
time you put your food in, stand watching it, stop it, stir
it (as microwaves tend to make everything gloop together),
then stare at it some more, I reckon my steamed veggies or
grilled chicken or boiled egg isn't far behind you! Is it also

really worth the saved seconds, when so much research is also coming out saying we should slow down and eat our food much, much more slowly for our health and digestion? It's a case, to me, of a false economy of time.

Microwave ready meals

Even though we can't say definitively whether microwaves are good or bad for you, their frequent companion – microwave meals – are definite bad guys for stacks of reasons. For a start, they're pre-cooked. Pre-cooking and reheating causes food to lose a whole load (if not almost all) of its nutritional value. The goodness of this energy-giving source is already depleted when you bought it, and will be depleted even more when you reheat it. These meals are packaged in plastic. Heated-up plastic is never going to be a healthy thing. Worst of all, they have a very high salt and sugar content, and are often stuffed full of other flavourings and chemicals to make them more palatable, extend their sell-by date and make them go brown or crispy without using an oven. Does that sound like the sort of fuel you want to charge your body with? Didn't think so.

I used to eat these things regularly when I was a soldier. Trust me: they never taste like they look on the packet and are a million miles away from a freshly cooked meal. They might be quick and convenient, but they're a nutritional nightmare. Stay away from them. Stay smart.

FASTING & DETOXING

I've fasted on several occasions. Sometimes it's been voluntary, sometimes it most definitely hasn't, when I've been stuck out in the wild with little to eat but insects! I've found this incredibly hard, but I've also found that it helped me to think more clearly, gave me an amazing energy boost, a sense of achievement and somehow brought me closer to nature.

On the other hand, fasting for too long has had the opposite effect and made me feel quite stressed out. When I did a combat-survival exercise as part of Special Forces training, I was on very limited rations – fewer than 300 calories a day for a two-week period, moving across mountains in winter, sleeping rough and being hunted by dogs and soldiers. It took its toll, but it was possible. On the other hand, on my TV show *The Island*, the contestants had very limited food for six weeks. They looked incredible living off just fish and coconuts!

For many people, fasting or going on a 'detox' are popular solutions to the problems of losing excess weight or gaining more energy. The question is: how healthy is this really?

What are fasting and detoxing?

A fast involves cutting out most food and reducing calorie intake to zero, or almost zero.

A detox involves consuming specific foods that help the body rid itself of toxins, as well as cutting out certain foods that put a strain on the body, such as alcohol, fried foods and sugar.

In reality, though, fasting and detoxing can be very similar, depending on which foods, and how much food, you decide to cut out.

An ancient tradition

When I'm in a survival situation, I never forget that the old ways, passed down by indigenous peoples over countless generations, and which have stood the test of time, are often the best.

Fasting is one of those. It has been observed in many cultures and religions for centuries. There is hardly a religion in the world that does not have fasting as one of its traditions. Many of our primitive ancestors fasted as well. I can't help thinking that something that has been practised for that long must have some benefit.

I've also noticed that when animals (both wild and domestic) get injured or ill, they will often fast for days or even weeks on end, consuming only small amounts of water as they let their bodies rest and recuperate. It's almost as if they know something we don't: that the body can heal much more quickly when we don't eat. It makes sense: if we give our digestion a break, our body can channel its resources into repair, recovery and detoxification.

Animals also sometimes fast during the mating season. Perhaps they look more attractive to the opposite sex once they've lost a few pounds!

The upsides of fasting and detoxing...

Fasting and detoxing give you numerous beneficial physical effects. You'll give your digestion a break (and for almost all of us, trust me, it needs it!), you'll help clear out excess toxins from your body, you'll lose some weight and you'll give your body a chance to heal and repair itself.

There can also be a number of positive mental effects. You might find you have a clearer mind, as you have more space and time to do other things. You'll learn to be grateful for the abundance of food we have available to us. You'll temporarily cut any emotional ties you might have with food and it can help you overcome addictions. And you'll begin to prepare the body for a generally healthier lifestyle.

What's more, if you feel great while fasting and terrible when going back to your normal diet, it may be a sign that certain foods or drinks you normally have don't agree with you. This is a fantastic opportunity to discover which foods are the culprits and to cut them out permanently, or at least for several months while your body recovers. Good examples of such foods are dairy, bread and coffee. They may be giving you symptoms that you didn't realize you had before fasting.

... and the downsides

Toxins are stored in fat cells, so when we lose weight while we fast they can end up in the bloodstream. This can give you several nasty side effects, such as headaches, nausea, mood swings or even an outbreak of spots on your face. You may also feel lightheaded or dizzy as your body adjusts to the lack of food. I tend to plan my fasts around days that aren't too busy or filled with important meetings (or photo shoots!).

How to do it

First things first: if you suffer from a medical condition, are on medication, are physically weakened, pregnant, breastfeeding or underweight, take professional medical advice before embarking on a fast or detox.

If not: give it a go!

As with most things, moderation is the key. One or two days of fasting could do you the world of good. Any longer than that and, like me, you might start to feel a negative effect. But everyone's different: some people will be comfortable fasting for longer, some people for less time. You should find out what suits you by dipping your toe in the water. Try drinking nothing but liquidized home-made vegetable soups for a day and seeing how you feel, before progressing to a water or vegetable-juice fast the following day. You could easily and safely do this every few weeks.

If you're the skinny, fast-burning type who feels the need to eat constantly and often feels cold, fasting on just water might be quite uncomfortable and stressful to your system. You may be better off sticking to warm vegetable soups and hot herbal teas for a couple of days. If you are the type that has tons of energy, a little excess weight and a naturally warmer body temperature, and you can skip a meal without feeling dizzy or panicky, fasting for several days on water, vegetable juices or raw salads may suit you perfectly well. Experiment, but in moderation. You will be healthier for it.

Make sure you always drink sufficient fluids if you're fasting. This will help kill your hunger and will also help flush out the toxins that may be released into your system.

And remember: it is better and easier to fast when it is warm outside than when it's cold. So fast in spring or summer, rather than in the middle of winter.

Detoxing supplements

There are many supplements and powders available on the market that claim to be detoxifying. Some of them work, some don't. Here are a few I'd be happy to use:

Milk thistle and dandelion – these are scientifically proven to support our liver's detoxification processes. Taking them in capsule or liquid form can certainly help during a fast or detox.

Probiotics – may help with rebalancing and restoring your digestion. Take in capsule or powder form.

Green powders – chlorella, spirulina and wheatgrass can have a cleansing and detoxifying effect while giving you an awesome energy boost.

However, once again, it is about moderation. You truly don't need (or want) a cupboard full of expensive, unproven supplements!

Don't fancy a fast? Here's the easy solution

Although fasts and detoxes can help you to feel more energetic, clean and lean in the short term, permanently changing the way you eat is a far cleverer solution – and not nearly so restrictive. If you follow my 8-week plan on page 233, you'll discover that it acts like a gentle but effective detox. You'll find yourself cutting out all the foods that many people have a hard time digesting, or which cause weight gain and sluggishness. It'll make you feel amazing and ready for anything – both physically and mentally. And ultimately, that's the goal.

SPORTS NUTRITION

Exercise and nutrition go hand in hand. You can't expect to exercise at optimal levels if you're not putting the right fuel in the tank.

Sports nutrition itself is a bit of a science, especially if you're a top athlete. But few of us realize the importance of nutrition in our simple day-to-day exercise regimes. Even if you attend the gym just twice a week, or occasionally go for a jog, what you eat *before* exercising and how you refuel *after* your session can literally make or break your body – and kill or kindle your motivation to exercise again.

Eating habits and motivation

People often quote their lack of self-discipline, their low fitness and energy levels or their lack of motivation as an excuse not even to begin to exercise or eat healthily. The good news is, those negative attributes are not who you really are. More often than not it is what you eat, or don't eat, that makes you feel this way and prevents you from making changes or performing at the level you're capable of.

It makes sense if you think about it. Fill a car with rubbish fuel and it'll never purr down the motorway. But let me give you some examples of things many of us have experienced during exercise. (And trust me, I've experienced them all myself at some point.)

◉ Just 5 minutes into your run you get a terrible stitch and think you must be the most unfit person ever!

Possible reason: A stitch is often caused by eating (even if it was healthily) too close to the start of your exercise session. It may have nothing to do with your fitness level at all.

● Despite endless training sessions, you just don't seem to be able to gain any muscle bulk or strength.

Possible reason: You keep missing that important muscle-rebuilding time-window straight after your exercise session, or you do refuel but use the wrong kinds of food.

● Instead of the exercise 'high' everybody always talks about, you experience an exercise 'low' following your workout. You feel drained and have to drag yourself though the remainder of the day.

Possible reason: You failed to refuel yourself properly with the correct foods and fluids *straight* after your exercise session. Your body is running on a low – and so is your mind!

● 10 minutes into your exercise class you run out of steam and can't give it 100 per cent. You can't wait for the class to be over!

Possible reason: You may not have fuelled up properly on the right carbohydrates and fluids a few hours before the class started. Your muscles have now quickly run out of their precious energy stores.

● You feel tired, sluggish, unmotivated and don't feel like exercising at all.

Possible reason: You haven't hydrated yourself well throughout the day. Low body fluids often result in sleepiness and lack of motivation. Sugary food, white flour products and other processed foods often have the same sluggish, de-motivating effect.

The solution to all the above issues can be as simple as knowing *when* and *what* to eat or drink. None of those reasons given can be defined as 'who you are' – they are simply a product of eating or drinking the wrong nutrition. That's where my exercise basics, my fuelling rules and my hydrating rules come in.

THREE EXERCISE BASICS

1. The main fuel your muscles use during exercise, especially during high-intensity workouts, is carbohydrate.

2. The secondary fuel your muscles use during exercise is fat, especially when you exercise at lower intensity for several hours at a time.

3. The main fuel your muscles need *after* exercise is protein, combined with some complex carbohydrates. This aids muscle recovery, muscle repair and repletes lost energy reserves.

BEAR'S FIVE EXERCISE FUELLING RULES

1. Don't starve yourself pre- or post-exercise. Even if you exercise in order to get rid of excess fat, *pre-fuelling* and *refuelling* with the *correct foods* are key to keeping your energy levels balanced during the session and for the remainder of the day. They are also key to helping reshape your body in the right places – more muscle, less fat.

2. Do not eat a full meal *less* than 2 hours before your session. If you plan a main meal before your workout, have this at least 2 to 4 hours before training. Exercising on a full or even semi-full stomach can be disastrous and lead to discomfort such as a stitch, breathlessness, muscle cramps or overall reduced performance. Even a healthy meal takes time to digest – especially when it contains protein, which is a slow-digesting food. Your stomach requires energy to break it down. This energy will be directed away from other parts of the body, such as the muscles, resulting in reduced performance and endurance.

3. Your main meal, several hours before the workout, should consist of a combination of lean proteins, complex carbohydrates and a little fat. All the breakfast, lunch and dinner recipes in the back of the book fit that bill perfectly. Choose anything, from a quick breakfast smoothie or a filling veggie soup with some of the protein-rich flourless bread on page 205, to a bowl of venison chilli or some grilled fish with sweet potato and vegetables.

4. If you have not eaten anything for more than 2–4 hours before your workout, at least opt for a small, easy-to-digest, carbohydrate-rich snack 45 minutes–1 hour before your workout. For example: a ripe banana or other piece of ripe fruit, a few dates, a fruit smoothie (without added protein or nuts), a small fruit and vegetable/ginger shake (beetroot is ideal!), or a juice. Your muscles can quickly run out of energy reserves if you train on an entirely unfuelled body.

5. Don't delay refuelling yourself after your workout. There is an important time-window, from immediately after you finish up to 45–90 minutes after training, when your muscles are most receptive to recovery, repair and strengthening. Eat an easy-to-digest protein- and carbohydrate-rich snack within this time-window. Examples are: Protein Bombs (pages 171, 172), Instant-energy Flapjacks (page 174), a slice of Banana Walnut Bread (page 181), one of my Post-workout Smoothies (page 226), or simply blend up a banana or mango with two scoops of protein powder and some almond milk.

Then, have a light, healthy meal containing protein and plenty of vegetables within 2 hours of your session. Vegetables are full of antioxidants and can help to reduce muscle aches and pains the next day.

BEAR'S FIVE EXERCISE HYDRATION TIPS

1. Beetroot juice is a great pre-exercise drink. Not only does it contain carbohydrates to fuel your muscles, beetroot also raises nitric oxide levels in your blood. This is excellent for cardiovascular function and muscle performance.

2. If you have a hard time giving up coffee, have your cup prior to your exercise session. That way, you can utilize its stimulating effect. However, you really don't want to become reliant on caffeine for performance, so use it sparingly. Nature will always guide you best. See the coffee section on pages 82–3.

3. Drink ½ litre of fluid up to 30 minutes before your workout, and at least ½ litre of fluid immediately after you finish. This is the safest rule for everyone, but remember that fluid loss will depend on the type of exercise (a casual jog versus a high-intensity tactical training class), the location of your exercise (outside in the sun versus an air-conditioned gym) and your fitness level. Take small sips of water at regular intervals throughout your session if it is a sweaty one. Do not drink big gulps of water during a session, as this can lead to gastrointestinal discomfort or a stitch. If you are exercising for more than an hour, after 30 minutes start sipping from a proper rehydration drink instead of just water. See 4 below for the recipe.

4. The best rehydration fluids don't just contain water but also electrolytes and some carbohydrates. During an intense workout you lose water, electrolytes and carbohydrates. I don't rely on sugary sports drinks to replace these. I make my own and it's super-simple and cheap. I either mix a pinch of quality salt with 2 tablespoons maple syrup and 2 tablespoons lemon juice in 1 pint water, or I have coconut water (naturally bursting with electrolytes) mixed with some fresh fruit juice, cherry juice concentrate or a piece of fresh fruit. Continue to rehydrate with water in the hours following your workout.

5. Plant foods can also keep you hydrated. Not only are they full of antioxidants that help to speed up recovery after exercise, but most fruit and vegetables contain water to help you stay hydrated much longer, making even hot yoga sweat sessions more bearable.

COCONUT OIL FOR ENERGY

You all know my love for coconut already. It's such an amazing, great-tasting survival superfood. Since swapping butter for coconut oil, I've found an increase in my energy and overall endurance, for good reasons. Coconut oil can be rapidly absorbed and converted into fuel, as I've explained in the chapter on fats (see page 33). Now I take chunks of coconut with me on long hikes or adventure races – it can be a lifesaver, and tastes delicious as a snack.

Fuelling yourself when you're out on the trail

Fuelling your body for long treks requires a slightly different approach to fuelling for short, intense workouts.

Without exception, all the breakfasts in the recipe section of this book are excellent pre-trail fuel. They provide a good combination of protein, complex carbohydrates and good fats, which will help you to keep going for quite a few hours.

You will need a similar combination of nutrients – proteins, fats and carbs – to help sustain you if you're out for a long time. Besides the simple but super-healthy choice of fresh or dried fruit with nuts and seeds, try the Chocolate Brownies (page 188), Instant-energy Flapjacks (page 174), Spicy Buckwheat Breakfast Muffins (page 120), Super-quick Fig and Pecan Energy Bars (page 173), Coconut Apricot Balls (page 182), Protein Bombs (page 171), Banana Walnut Bread (page 181) or Indian Quinoa Bites (page 178). They are all packed with nutrients and energy, and they also taste great. Don't underestimate this. Napoleon said that an army marches on its stomach, and he was right – sometimes we need motivation to keep going. Energy-giving fuel that also tastes great can really provide that.

Sports supplements

I don't take supplements to enhance performance, fat loss or muscle growth. I have tried several in the past. Some may have helped, but I found their effectiveness hard to measure. I preferred to find out what I could naturally achieve from a workout by relying on the capabilities of my body when fuelled with the correct food. The results were great. I much prefer always to seek out knowledge about how to maximize what nature has given us to thrive and perform. This is about natural food and natural training, and it is no surprise that we then get a body that is natural-looking: lean, in proportion and toned. Just as nature intended! Trust nature, not drugs, and know that shortcuts always have a pay-off and the downsides can be massive.

The closest thing to a sports supplement I will have is protein powder, which is just so easy to mix into smoothies for a quick post-workout protein fix.

SHOPPING PRINCIPLES

Nobody wants shopping for food to be a drag. Nobody wants to traipse around trying to find obscure, expensive ingredients. My life's too busy for that, and I bet yours is too.

So how do we make sure, when we go shopping, that we're buying the right stuff to put in our bodies to fuel it properly and to increase our chances of longevity and vitality?

Well, one way is to arm ourselves with the information in this book. I hope that by the time you've got to the end, you'll look at food in a better, healthier way.

The second way is to learn how to read ingredients.

Less is more

When it comes to ingredients, a very simple rule of thumb applies: less is more. It's likely that the fewer ingredients a product contains, the more nutritional value it has. Although there may be some exceptions, generally if a food contains five or more ingredients it is unlikely to be fully natural or 100 per cent healthy. If something contains a list of ingredients you've never even heard of, with complicated-sounding names that are hard to pronounce and probably even harder to digest, it's best just to leave it on the shelf.

To show you what I mean, let's compare two breakfast products. One contains a single ingredient, the other contains more than twenty.

Oats

This is a simple breakfast that many of us enjoy for its warming, filling and energy-giving properties.

Ingredients: oats!

This one ingredient contains a whole range of amazing nutrients. Below I have named a few and briefly given a description of their function in the body, just to help you understand their importance.

Calcium – important for healthy teeth, bones, fluid balance, muscle contractions, blood clotting, heart health, nerve impulses and the secretion of breast milk.

Iron – necessary for transporting oxygen around the body, the production of energy, proper enzyme function and the metabolism of other vitamins and minerals.

Beta-glucans – excellent for the removal of excess cholesterol in the digestive tract as well as supporting immune function.

Unrefined carbohydrates – a great source of 'slow-release' energy.

Vitamin B1 – necessary for cardiovascular and nervous-system health and for the normal development of the brain.

Vitamin B3 – necessary for energy production, a healthy nervous system, healthy skin, the production of sex hormones and the removal of bad cholesterol from the blood.

Vitamin B5 – important for energy production, growth of new cells, healthy skin and hair, immunity and hormone balance.

Vitamin B6 – good for skin, the nervous system and brain function; fights premature ageing, enhances immunity and helps to protect against heart disease.

Folate – necessary for the formation of our DNA and healthy development of the human embryo.

Magnesium – vital for normal muscle and heart function, healthy bones and teeth, nervous-system function, healthy blood pressure, fluid balance and proper immune function.

Potassium – supports our muscles, heart and nervous system, and helps to maintain healthy fluid balance.

Zinc – involved in energy production, immune function, healthy skin, sexual development and the health of our reproductive organs.

Chromium – regulates blood-sugar balance, which is important in the prevention of diabetes.

Antioxidants – help prevent premature ageing and protect us from the development of diseases such as cancer and heart disease.

Essential fats – vital for the growth and maintenance of our brain, heart and skin, for hormone balance and immunity.

All the above are naturally contained within this one, simply packaged, practically unprocessed grain.

Breakfast cereal
Now, we'll take a fictional but realistic box of 'high-fibre, low-fat', scrumptious-looking breakfast cereal flakes, with Bursting Berry flavour and added vitamins and minerals.

Ingredients: wheat, sugar, toasted oats, soya bean oil, flavoured apples (2 per cent apples, artificial flavour and colour, sodium sulfite), high fructose corn syrup, salt, partially hydrogenated palm kernel oil, non-fat dry milk, whey, corn syrup solids, confectioner's glaze, humectant (glycerol), natural and artificial flavours, cinnamon, reduced iron, riboflavin (B2), vitamin A palmitate, folic acid, vitamin B12.

Some breakfast cereals have even longer lists. And although I'm known for eating some pretty weird stuff, even I draw the line at all that!

Granted, not all the ingredients on the list are bad. This breakfast cereal does contain oats and even a small percentage of what was once fruit (before it entered the processing factory). However, the majority of ingredients are there to add crunch, texture, sweetness, saltiness, colour, flavour, smell, or as an aid to keep the flake together in its fancy shape. (You don't need me to tell you that Mother Nature does not grow berry-flavoured crunchy flakes.) If the second or third ingredient is sugar, don't even consider feeding this to your kids!

During the manufacturing of this cereal – which involves heating, mixing, pressing all the ingredients together, adding preservatives to extend shelf life, and packaging – most of the vitamins and minerals are lost. Therefore, at the end of this lengthy process, to ensure there is at least *something* healthy left in the final product, these lost vitamins and minerals have been added again, in a chemical form that is usually not very well recognized or usable by the human body (more on this on page 87).

By the way, did you notice the lack of actual berries in the 'berry-flavoured' cereal? This is common. Products with a certain flavour often don't contain the actual product.

Right now is a good moment to grab some cans, boxes and pre-packed food from your storage cupboards, fridge or freezer and read their lists of ingredients. Take a moment to note down those ingredients you don't immediately recognize and look them up online. Are they healthy? Are they natural? Are they dangerous? This will raise your awareness of what you are actually eating.

This awareness is the first step to re-educating yourself about the daily food choices you will make for energy, longevity and maximum health.

So here they are. My shopping rules. Think of them as a supermarket survival guide!

BEAR'S 10 SHOPPING SURVIVAL RULES

1. Choose items that look and are as unprocessed as possible. Think: oats, nuts, seeds, fruits, vegetables, herbs, brown rice, beans and pulses and clean-cut, unprocessed organic meat and fish.

2. Choose products with packaging that makes few or no health claims. Avoid those claiming to be 'low-fat', 'sugar-free', 'with added vitamins', 'zero-calorie' and so on.

3. Choose products that have fewer than five ingredients listed – or no ingredients listed at all (like fresh fruit and vegetables) and certainly no ingredients you can't pronounce.

4. Don't choose foods that have wheat, sugar or dairy as their main ingredient. Watch out for sugar disguised under different names.

5. Check the total sugar content of a product, remembering that 4 grams of sugar equal 1 teaspoon.

6. Don't choose foods you saw in a TV advert. Healthy foods don't need advertising.

7. Don't go for 'instant' or 'fried' foods or pre-packed ready-made meals, and use condiments sparingly – only to add a little extra flavour to your fresh meals.

8. Don't be fooled by foods labelled 'Part of your 5 -a-day'. Many processed foods carry this label, but they aren't necessarily healthy. According to packaging claims, you could get your '5-a-day' from tinned pasta in tomato sauce, frozen lollipops, baked beans, a frozen ready meal and a carton of fruit juice. None of this would provide you with real nutrition, just with tons of sugar and salt. Foods that *properly* add to your '5-a-day' are often not labelled as such: fruit, vegetables, seeds, nuts, beans, lean protein and other real foods.

9. Sometimes you need to be as observant in everyday life as you are in the wild. Healthier or more obscure or natural products (quinoa, for example) aren't always placed at eye level. Make sure to look at the top and bottom of the supermarket shelves when you shop. You may find a whole range of products you never knew your supermarket stocked!

10. Supermarkets aren't your only shopping option. Don't shy away from visiting local farm shops or from shopping online – which can be much cheaper and offer much more (organic) choice than your local supermarket. Health shops can be an absolute treasure chest and can help you discover a whole range of new, healthy foods to add to your daily diet.

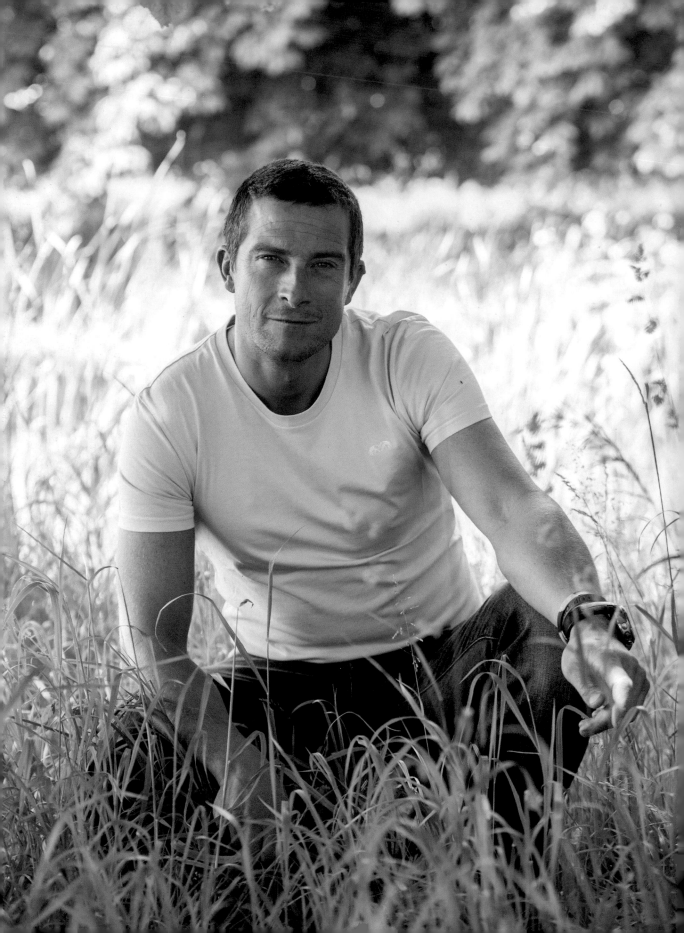

THE
FUEL

THE LARDER

Did you know that on average people have no more than about twenty standard items of food in their kitchen and pretty much buy the same ingredients each week! This book is all about expanding the content of your kitchen staples and your day-to-day food choices.

Here are the items I always make sure to have in my larder or fridge and which will help you on your way to creating healthy breakfasts, lunches, dinners and snacks.

⊙ Oats (opt for steel-cut oats if you can) ⊙ Quinoa ⊙ Almond flour ⊙ Buckwheat flour ⊙ Coconut flour ⊙ Protein powder (hemp, rice or pea, or a mix) ⊙ Organic brown basmati rice ⊙ Several tins of beans and chickpeas

⊙ Nuts and seeds (almost all varieties available) ⊙ Nut butters such as almond, cashew or peanut butter without added salt or sugar

⊙ Coconut oil ⊙ Extra-virgin olive oil ⊙ Hemp oil ⊙ Apple cider vinegar ⊙ Sun-dried tomatoes ⊙ Tomato paste ⊙ Olives ⊙ Marmite ⊙ Mustard ⊙ Curry paste (fresh, frozen or from a jar) ⊙ Nutritional yeast flakes ⊙ Organic stock cubes or powder

⊙ Berries (fresh or frozen) ⊙ Apples ⊙ Bananas ⊙ Dried whole dates, figs and apricots ⊙ Whole coconuts ⊙ Lemons and limes ⊙ Ginger

⊙ Stevia ⊙ Maple syrup ⊙ Baobab powder ⊙ Lucuma powder ⊙ Raw unsweetened cacao powder ⊙ Vanilla extract

⊙ Green veggies: think cucumber, spinach, broccoli, kale, rocket, leek, celery, etc ⊙ Garlic and onions ⊙ Avocados ⊙ Carrots ⊙ (Chilli) peppers ⊙ Tomatoes ⊙ Sweet potatoes ⊙ Frozen peas and other frozen veg

⊙ Almond, oat, coconut, hemp or rice milk ⊙ Coconut cream

⊙ Organic free-range eggs ⊙ Frozen game (mostly venison and buffalo) ⊙ Fresh or frozen fish (anything you fancy)

⊙ Basil ⊙ Thyme ⊙ Rosemary ⊙ Coriander ⊙ Mint ⊙ Selection of dried herbs and spices (see page 68)

⊙ Pink Himalayan crystal salt ⊙ Black peppercorns (in grinder)

⊙ Beetroot juice ⊙ Coconut water

The following recipes have been carefully put together to ensure you can fuel yourself with a variety of meals and snacks, each of which tastes fantastic, as well as helping you and your family take positive, life-enhancing steps towards fitter, leaner, more productive lives. That's the goal here.

This is how I eat and how my family eats – delicious recipes packed with health-promoting nutrients.

These recipes are a carefully crafted mix of our own creations and others we've adapted from delicious, healthy dishes across the globe. As with any recipes, feel free to adapt them to your own liking. Swap ingredients around, and never give up after the first try. We didn't!

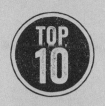

Kitchen tools
Blender
Food processor
Nut grinder
Loaf tin
Cake tin
Baking tray/dish
Brownie tin
Muffin tin
Box grater or spiralizer
A set of quality knives

NOTE

◎ When we say 'salt' we mean a good-quality unrefined salt (see page 47).

◎ Where a recipe calls for olive oil, use a good-quality extra-virgin type.

◎ When a recipe calls for coconut oil, we mean organic, raw, virgin coconut oil in solid form. The instructions will then tell you whether to melt it or not.

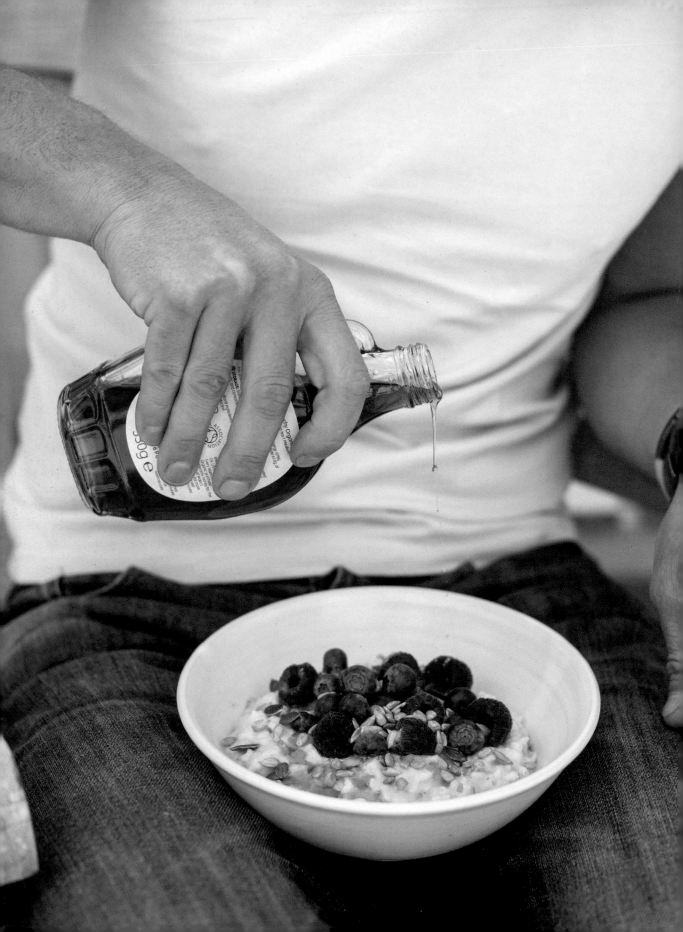

BREAKFASTS

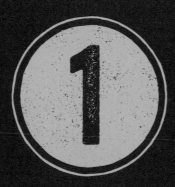

Seriously: ditch your sugary cereal or toast with jam. Choose an awesome breakfast smoothie or my Bear-style oats instead. Or turn your unhealthy weekend fry-up into a super-healthy feast. You can pack in a massive load of your daily vitamin and mineral intake by doing just that. It sets the tone for the rest of the day, and if you can't avoid a less healthy lunch or dinner, at least you've already done yourself a world of good before the day's even started.

BG SUPER-HEALTHY
SAUSAGES

Per person

1 chicken breast

1 medium zesty apple, chopped

½ thin leek, sliced

1 large garlic clove, skinned

a large handful of fresh mixed herbs (basil/ thyme/oregano, coriander/marjoram, parsley/chives or rosemary/thyme)

salt and pepper, to taste

olive oil for frying

I like a fry-up just as much as the next person, but they don't have to be greasy or unhealthy. Try this super-healthy one – it's loaded with protein and fresh veggies. Guaranteed to fill you up and deliver that positive protein hit!

Put all the ingredients in a food processor and process until you have a fine, mince-like mixture.

Use your hands to form the mixture into 4–6 sausage shapes and press them down so they are flat and about 1cm thick (this ensures that they get cooked through properly).

Either heat the olive oil in a pan and fry the sausages for several minutes on both sides until browned and cooked through; or preheat the oven to 200°C/400°F/gas mark 6, put the sausages on a lightly oiled baking sheet and bake them for 20 minutes, turning occasionally.

To complete your breakfast, serve with a poached egg, some grilled tomatoes and mushrooms and a slice of flourless bread (page 205). Baked beans optional!

You can make these sausages in batches and freeze them. The mixture also makes an awesome burger.

POWER PANCAKES

Makes about 6

130g buckwheat flour
200ml unsweetened
    almond milk
100ml water
½ tsp vanilla extract
½ tsp cinnamon
½ tsp salt
a dash of stevia (optional)
a little coconut oil for frying

Despite its deceptive name, buckwheat is entirely wheat- and gluten-free. Packed with protein and very filling, these pancakes will get you on the road, fast. They're awesome with some sliced banana or fresh berries and a sprinkle of flax seeds. Or with apples sautéed in cinnamon and a drizzle of maple syrup.

Mix all the ingredients together into a smooth batter using an electric mixer or hand whisk.

Melt a little coconut oil in a small, non-stick frying pan over medium heat. Add several large spoonfuls of the batter to the pan, tilting the pan from side to side to spread out the batter as thinly and evenly as possible.

Cook until the pancake can be lifted from the pan with a palette knife or spatula and the underside is a pale golden colour: this will take several minutes (as these pancakes don't have any egg, you'll need to cook them for a bit longer than regular pancakes). Flip the pancake over and cook the second side in the same way.

Transfer each pancake to a warm plate while you cook the rest of the batch. Serve while warm.

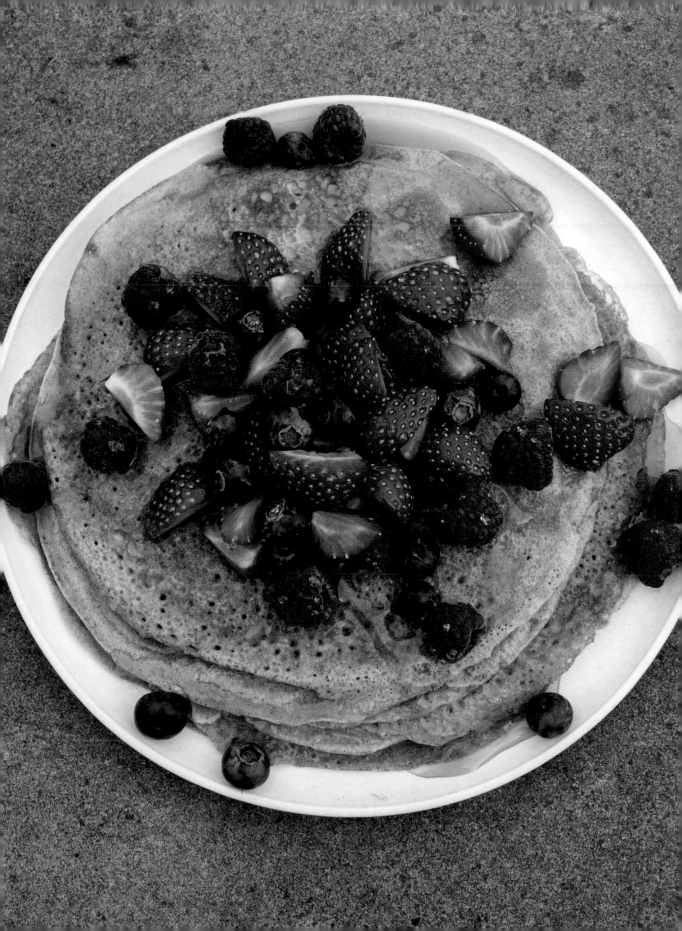

EGG MUFFINS

Makes 6

Approx. 6 small handfuls
  vegetables – choose from
  whatever you have in
  the fridge, but some great
  combos are: spinach,
  tomato and chive; kale,
  garlic and sun-dried
  tomato; spring onion and
  grated carrot; red onion
  and kale; red pepper and
  coriander; rocket and red
  onion; asparagus and
  broccoli; basil and tomato
6 eggs, beaten
salt and pepper
a little coconut or olive oil
  to grease the muffin tin

Optional extras

leftover cooked meat,
  chopped into very
  small pieces
thin slices of olive
thin slices of jalapeño
  pepper

Simple but tasty egg bites which can be made in any flavour you or your family like.

Preheat the oven to 175°C/350°F/gas mark 4. Line a 6-hole muffin tin with paper muffin cases.

Chop or finely grate your vegetables of choice, plus any optional extras, and put in a large bowl. Mix in the eggs and seasoning and stir to combine into a smooth batter.

Divide the mixture evenly between the muffin cases and bake for 20 minutes, or until a toothpick inserted in the centre of a muffin comes out clean.

Remove from the tin and cool slightly on a wire rack.

ALTERNATIVE: You can use this recipe to make two large omelettes. Blitz all the ingredients in a blender. Heat a little coconut or olive oil in a frying pan, pour in half the mixture and cook until the mixture is set. Remove from the pan and keep warm while you cook the remaining half.

FRUITY CHIA
POWER BOWL

Per person

3–4 tbsp chia seeds
250ml almond or
    coconut milk
a sprinkle of cinnamon
¼ mango, chopped into
    small chunks (other
    sweet fruits such as
    banana or a ripe pear
    are great too)

Busy morning ahead? No time to make breakfast? Spend just 3 minutes the night before making this simple and energizing power bowl. It's full of fibre, omega-3 oils, vitamins and minerals. It's filling and super-quick to make. If you've never tried chia seeds before, you may be quite surprised by their consistency once they've been soaked. Shara thinks it looks like frogspawn – but don't worry, it certainly doesn't taste like it with this recipe!

Mix all the ingredients together in a breakfast bowl with a whisk. Leave to soak for 30 minutes – or overnight – stirring it occasionally so you don't get clumps.

BEAR-STYLE OATS

Per person, choose from

2 tbsp mixed seeds (flax, pumpkin, sesame or sunflower) and a large handful of fresh berries

a small chopped semi-ripe banana, 1 tbsp organic peanut butter (no added sugar or salt) and a dash of cinnamon

1 tsp raw cacao powder, 1 small chopped semi-ripe banana, a small handful of cashew nuts and 2 tsp desiccated coconut

6 walnuts, 1 small cubed apple and a dash of cinnamon

a dash of maple syrup and a small handful of blanched almonds

Oats don't need to be boring – you can make yours taste different every day! Cook your oats in the usual way, according to the instructions on the packet, but use almond, coconut, hemp or oat milk instead of cows milk. Now add any of the ingredients on the left to help sustain you even longer and give you that winning extra nutrient boost.

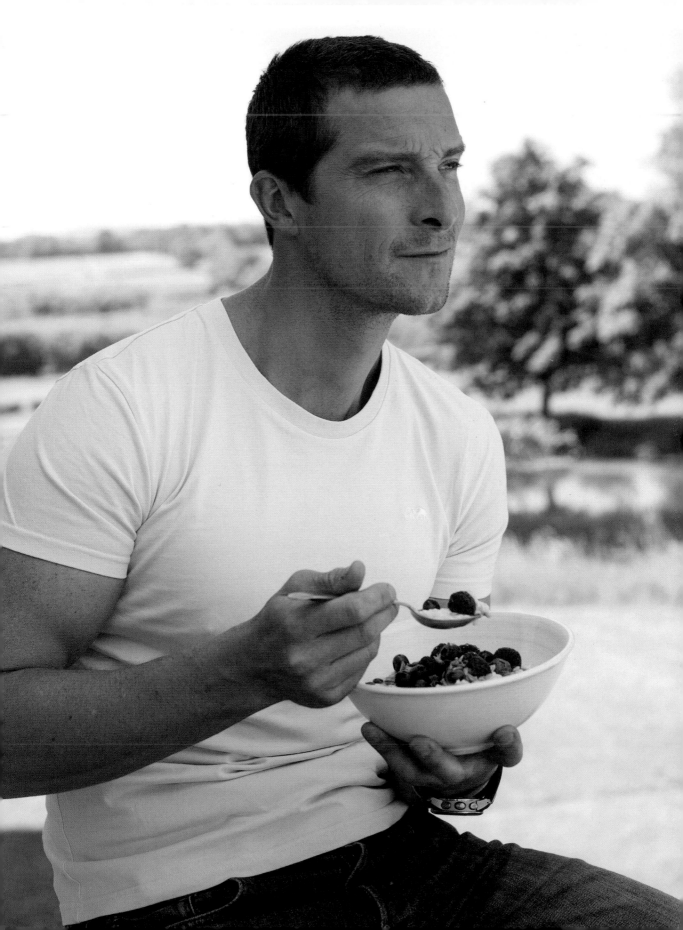

SPICY BUCKWHEAT
BREAKFAST MUFFINS

Makes 6–8

3–4 very ripe bananas,
    mashed to a purée
200g buckwheat flour
50g oats
80g chopped walnuts
25g (about 4 heaped tsp)
    ground flax seed
    (see page 71)
2 tsp baking powder
1 tsp baking soda
½ tsp sea salt
2 tsp cinnamon
1 tsp ginger powder
⅓ tsp ground black pepper
2 tbsp coconut oil, melted
2 tsp vanilla essence
100g carrots (about
    2 medium ones), grated
4 tbsp raisins (to taste),
    soaked in water for
    10 minutes
150–200ml coconut milk

These guys are *filling*. Brilliant as a quick breakfast, or to take with you while you're out and about.

Preheat the oven to 190°C/375°F/gas mark 5. Line 8 holes of a muffin tin with paper muffin cases, or lightly oil a 22cm cake tin and line it with lightly greased baking paper.

Using an electric mixer or a hand whisk, mix all the ingredients together, adding enough coconut milk to give you a thick batter.

Divide the mixture evenly between the muffin tins, filling them almost to the top, or spoon it all into the cake tin.

Bake for 20–25 minutes, or until a toothpick inserted in the centre comes out clean. Turn out of the tin and allow to cool on a wire rack.

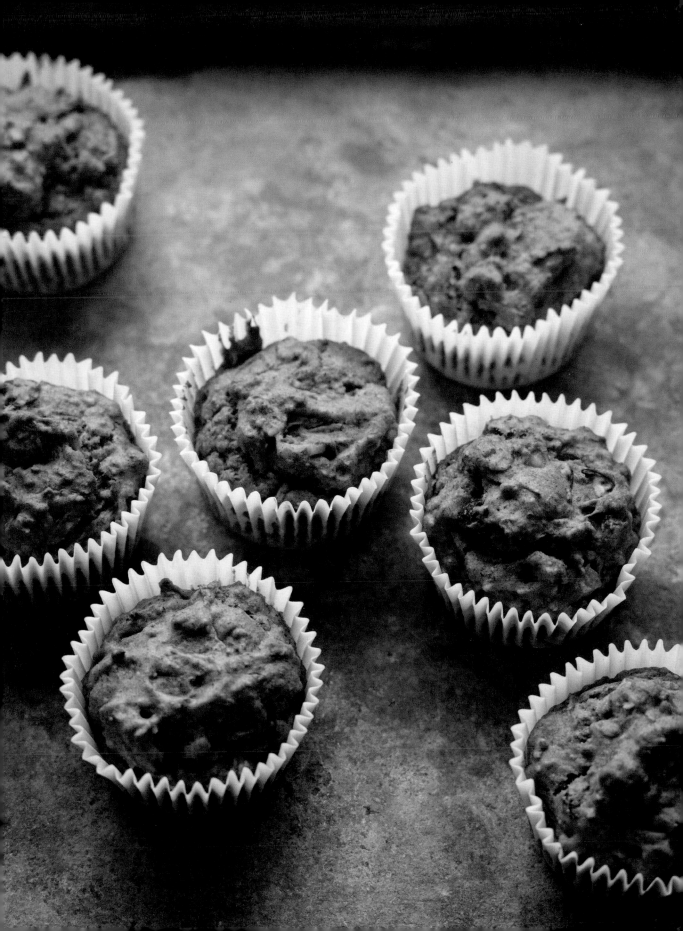

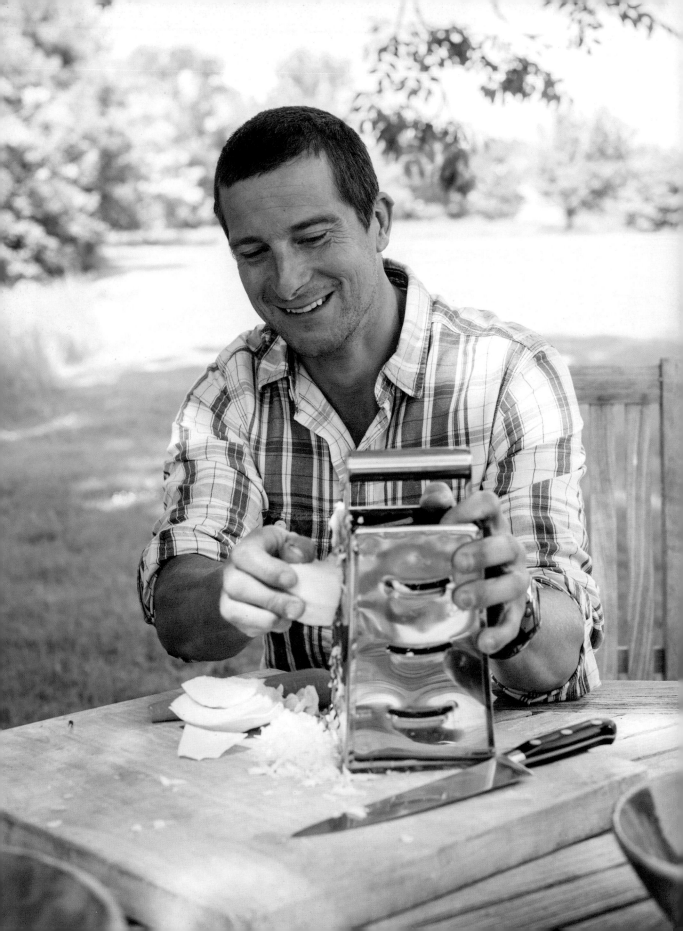

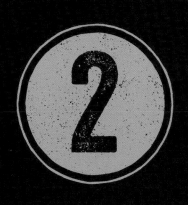

SALADS & LIGHT MEALS

2

You might have heard the expression 'Breakfast like a king, lunch like a prince, dine like a pauper.' Well, it has science behind it. As the day wears on, our digestion starts to relax, unwind and detoxify. It's much healthier to have a bigger lunch and a smaller dinner. This batch of recipes fits the bill. Eat light, feel light.

SHREDDED
SPROUT SALAD

Serves 2

300g Brussels sprouts
   (pick the largest ones you
   can find), finely grated
1 small to medium sweet
   but zesty apple, finely
   grated
1 tbsp maple syrup
1 tbsp apple cider vinegar
¼ tsp cinnamon
pinch of salt and a little
   freshly ground pepper
10 walnut halves, crushed
   into smaller pieces

I despised Brussels sprouts for years. The smell, the taste, the soggy consistency and the bloated feeling they caused. But that was probably because I only ever had them boiled to a pulp! This salad has made me love sprouts. Quick, easy, and you'd never guess my all-time least favourite vegetable is the main ingredient!

Cut off the outer leaves and tough stem from your Brussels sprouts and grate the sprouts using a box-grater (watch your fingers) or mandoline. Grate the apple, and add to the sprouts. Add all the remaining ingredients and mix well.

NOT YOUR AVERAGE
COLESLAW

**Serves 3 as a generous
    side dish**

¼ white cabbage

1 medium carrot

2 tbsp olive oil

1 tbsp wholegrain mustard

50g walnuts

1 tbsp maple syrup

1 tbsp lemon juice

seeds from ½ medium
    pomegranate

a handful of chopped
    coriander (optional)

**No mayonnaise needed, just fresh, crunchy, zesty
ingredients. Makes for a vitamin-packed side dish
– or you could do as I often do on 'lean' or 'fasting'
days and grab a big bowl for lunch.**

Grate the cabbage and carrot with a box-grater (or chop
them finely using a food processor). Transfer to a large
bowl and add all the other ingredients, mixing until they
are thoroughly combined.

This dish is best served cold, letting the flavours settle
in the fridge for about 30 minutes.

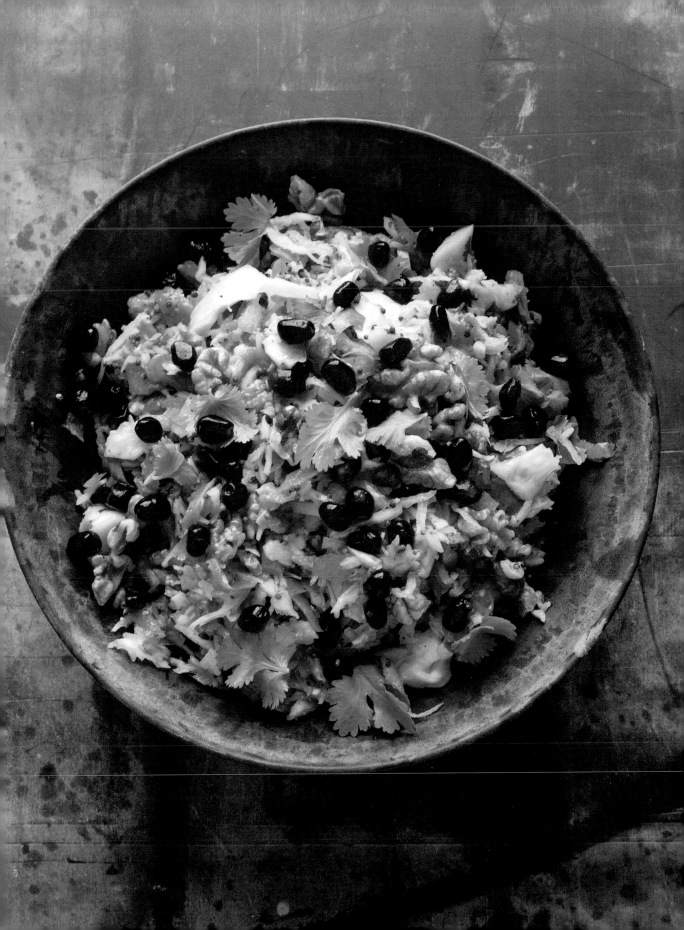

HIGH-ENERGY SALAD

Serves 2–3
200g quinoa
12 dried apricots,
   or 6 fresh ones
   (peaches work
   well too)
2 spring onions
2 large handfuls of rocket
   (about 50g)
50g peeled pistachios
   (other nuts such as
   walnuts or pecans
   are also good)
4 tbsp olive oil
2 tbsp lemon juice
30g golden raisins
salt and lots of fresh
   black pepper

Make this in big batches so you can add it to other meals as desired, or have it as a snack to fuel yourself easily.

Boil the quinoa in water with a little salt according to the instructions on the packet. Transfer to a large bowl.

In the meantime, finely chop the apricots, spring onions and rocket. Mix in with the quinoa, then stir in all the other ingredients.

This is delicious either hot or cold.

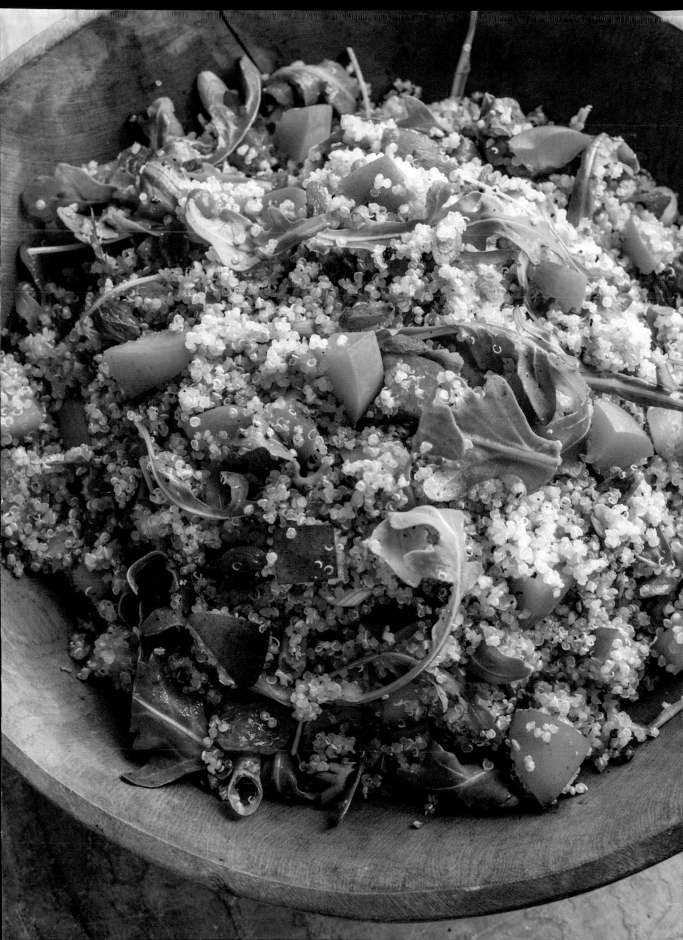

RAINBOW SALAD

Per person

Approx. 5 of the following:
broccoli, carrot, peppers,
cauliflower, cabbage,
courgettes, cress, curly
kale, tomatoes,
mushrooms, green
beans, sugar snap peas,
green asparagus tips,
basil, celery, fennel,
beetroot, sweet potato,
coriander, rocket, lettuce
leaves, spinach, leek,
spring onion.

For example, a combination
of 5 could be: several
broccoli florets, ¼ red
pepper, a small beetroot,
a large handful of rocket
and a carrot

Always add

½ garlic clove, skinned
and very finely chopped
¼ small red onion, skinned
and very finely chopped

Optional

olive oil
lemon juice
sea salt and freshly ground
black pepper
extra fresh herbs, to taste

When people think of salad, they often think of lettuce, tomato and cucumber. I certainly always used to. But almost any vegetable that can be eaten raw can taste great in a salad, provided it is chopped or grated small enough! That's the secret to a good salad with lots of variety – no one likes to eat big chunks of raw broccoli or beetroot. This salad is a real health bomb. The more colours you include, the more diverse the health benefits you'll get. Again, you can make big batches and serve it as a side to any meal, or have a bowl as a quick snack or light lunch.

Chop, or preferably grate, the vegetables as small as you can (I'm talking really tiny) and put them in a bowl. Mix in the garlic and onion. If you wish, add a pinch of sea salt, freshly ground pepper, a little olive oil, lemon juice and/or fresh herbs to taste. You can add some chopped olives, sun-dried tomatoes and jalapeno pepper slices for extra flavour.

This colourful salad also makes an excellent base for adding other ingredients, which turns it into a complete meal. You could use: a piece of grilled chicken or fish flaked into small pieces, a handful of cooked prawns, ½ chopped avocado, a handful of nuts or seeds, a coffee cup of beans or some cooked quinoa, ½ cup sprouted seeds, beans or lentils, or 2 tbsp freshly made dip such as hummus or guacamole.

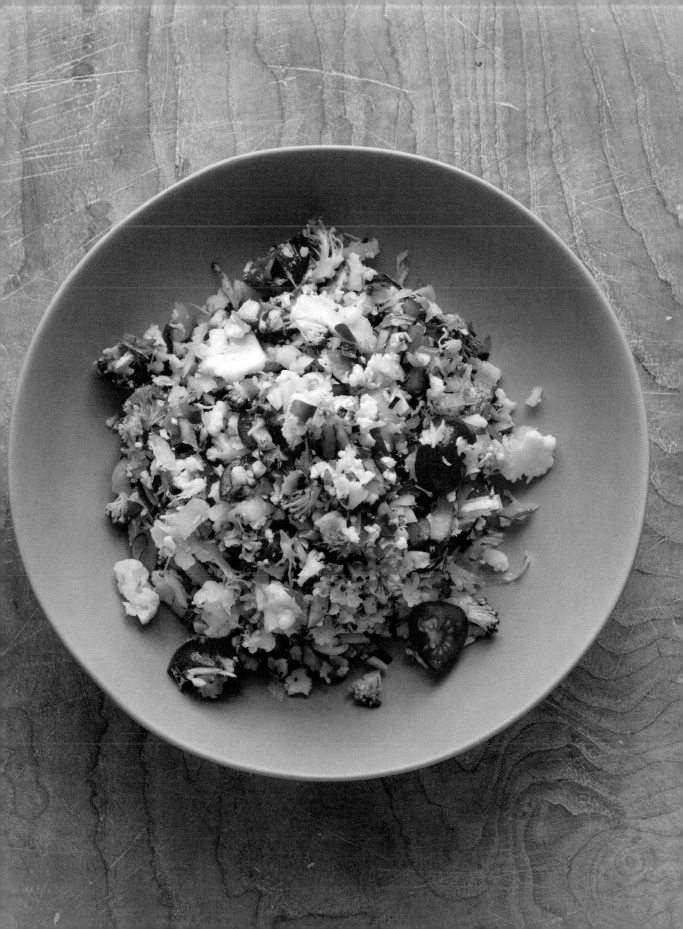

VITALITY VEG

Per person

vegetables (preferably
   green) of your choice
   (e.g. ½ leek, a few
   broccoli florets,
   2 handfuls of spring
   greens, ¼ red onion –
   just whatever veg you
   have in your fridge)
olive oil
salt and pepper
sun-dried tomatoes,
   chopped
chilli (fresh, dried or slices
   from a jar), to taste
1–2 tbsp nutritional yeast
salt and freshly ground
   pepper

**If you feel you need to catch up on your vegetable
intake, or if you are headed out for a cheat dinner
or party later, get your vegetables in beforehand.
This spicy veg bowl is simple, filling, tasty and
sorts all your vitamin needs.**

Steam your vegetables for about 5 minutes until tender.
Transfer to a bowl.

Add a generous drizzle of olive oil and all the other
ingredients. Mix thoroughly and get it down you while
it's hot. Job done.

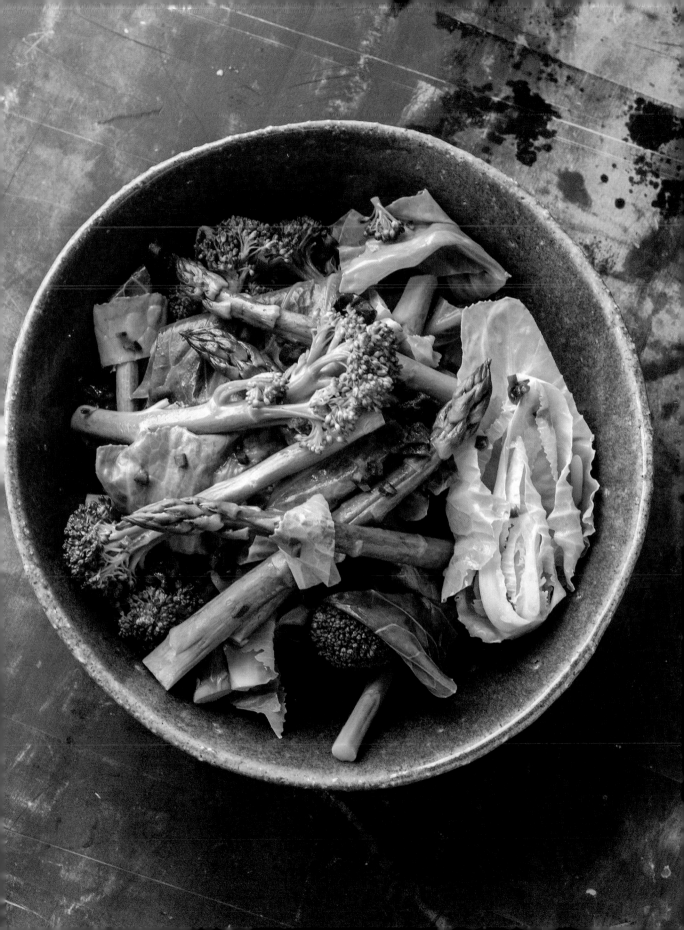

LIME AND CHILLI
CEVICHE

Serves 2–3

500g firm white fish (sea bass, sole, halibut or red snapper work well, but you can also use fresh shrimp or prawns)

1 tsp salt

freshly squeezed juice of 6 limes (don't squeeze too long and hard – you don't want any bitterness from the rind to come out)

½ bird's-eye chilli, deseeded and finely chopped (use more or less, depending on how hot you like it)

1 tsp finely chopped coriander

½ red onion, skinned, very finely sliced and briefly rinsed in water.

cherry tomatoes, chopped and deseeded

I've eaten all kinds of raw food in the wild. I'll be honest – some of it tastes better than others. But I first ate this raw fish dish in Ecuador many years ago. It's now a staple for me every time I am anywhere near South or Central America, but I also eat it at home as it is so easy to make. (By the way, the fish isn't *really* raw. It's 'cooked' in lime juice and perfectly safe.)

Cut your fish into chunks and put them in a non-metal dish. Rub them with the salt – it might seem a lot, but most of it will stay behind in the liquid.

Add the lime juice, chilli and coriander and mix with your hands. Sprinkle the red onion over the top, cover and put in the fridge.

If you like your fish fairly raw, you can eat this after about 10 minutes, which is just enough time for the lime juice to cook the outside of the fish. If you do this, make sure your fish is *incredibly* fresh – you don't want food poisoning. My family like their fish properly cooked through, so I leave it to sit for about 3 hours.

Serve with the cherry tomatoes on top, and a little more freshly chopped coriander, if you like.

At heart, I keep my ceviche super-simple, but once you've got the hang of how it's done you can add other things like chopped spring onion, celery, finely diced peppers or some grated ginger. In South America, I've had this served with slices of grapefruit, sweet potato and avocado. What a great combination!

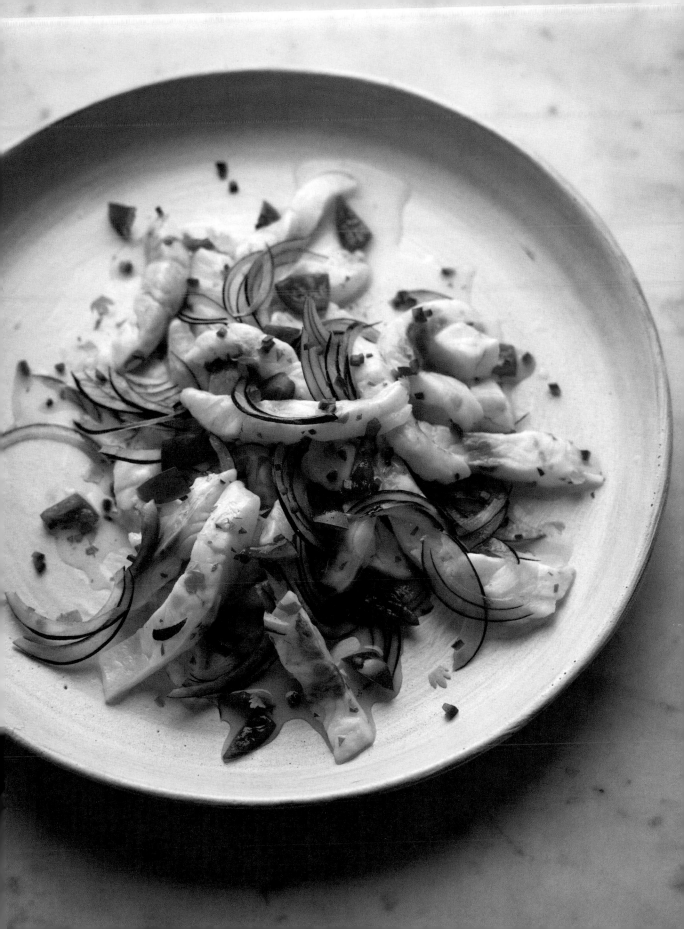

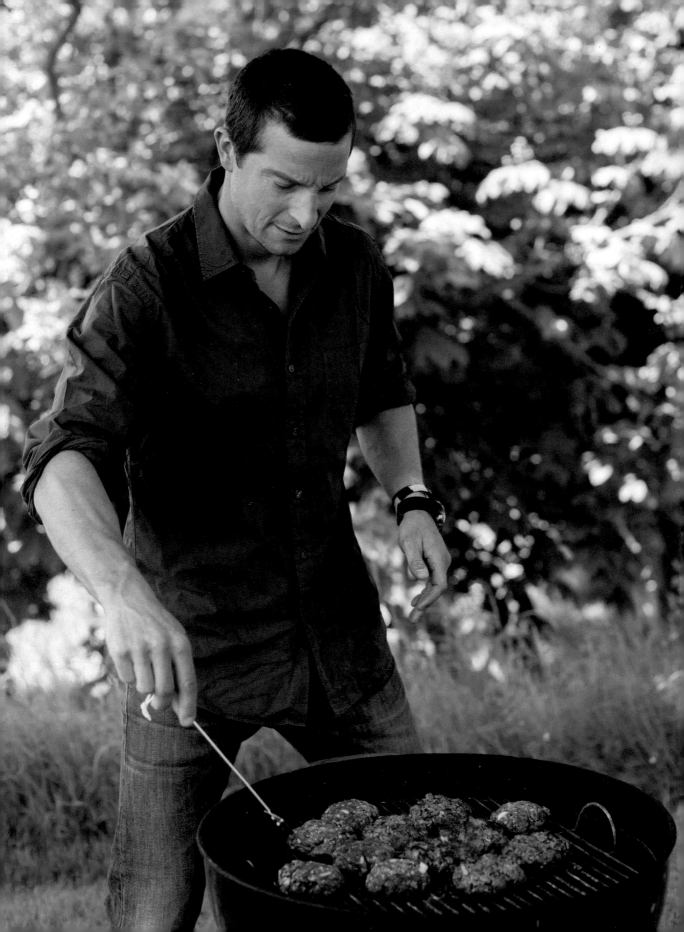

MAIN MEALS

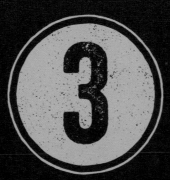

When we change the way we eat, it's the comfort foods and old favourites we miss the most. But I don't want you to feel like you're missing out on anything. Here we've re-created some of our favourite meals using only wholesome ingredients. These recipes are healthy and filling, yet give you that old familiarity of comfort food.

SOUTH INDIAN CHICKEN

Serves 2

2 organic, free-range
chicken breasts
sea salt and lots and
lots of black pepper
1 tbsp coconut oil
or olive oil
2.5cm piece of ginger,
very finely chopped
4 garlic cloves, skinned
and finely chopped
1 onion, skinned and
finely sliced
1 tsp turmeric
2 tomatoes, finely diced
a small handful of fresh
coriander leaves

Simple, flavoursome, easy: my kind of recipe.

Cut the chicken breasts into 4 pieces. Season with a *lot* of pepper (it's part of the recipe, not just a bit of seasoning) and some salt.

Heat some coconut or olive oil in a pan and brown the chicken, turning it a few times to ensure a good colour. Remove the chicken from the pan. Add ginger, garlic, onion and turmeric to the pan and fry for a couple of minutes. Add the tomatoes and a couple of tablespoons of water. Cover, turn down the heat and simmer for 2 minutes.

Put the chicken back into the pan, cover again and cook until tender. Stir in the coriander leaves. Add a little more pepper and salt if it needs it.

Serve accompanied by salad or steamed vegetables.

VENISON SHEPHERD'S PIE

Serves 4

For the topping
800g peeled, diced sweet
  potato (approx. 2 large
  sweet potatoes)
1 tbsp olive oil
1 tbsp coconut oil
1 tbsp chopped rosemary
salt and pepper

For the filling
500g venison, cubed
2 tbsp olive oil, plus
  a little extra
1 medium onion, skinned
  and diced
1 stalk celery, diced
2 medium carrots, diced
150g cauliflower, chopped
  into very small florets
4 garlic cloves, skinned
  and finely chopped
5 chestnut mushrooms,
  sliced
1 heaped tbsp tomato paste
1 vegetable stock cube
1 tsp chopped rosemary
1 tbsp Worcestershire
  sauce (or tamari sauce
  if you want to be
  gluten-free)
125ml water
¼ tsp cinnamon
salt and black pepper
frozen peas

Home-made venison mince (don't worry, this takes less than 2 minutes to make) is what makes this shepherd's pie really stand out. This dish is lean, clean, honest, full of fresh vegetables and incredibly tasty.

Preheat the oven to 200°C/400°F/gas mark 6.

First, make the topping. Cover the sweet potatoes with water and boil for about 5 minutes until softened. Drain, then add the remaining topping ingredients. Mash with a potato masher and set aside.

Now for the filling. Put the diced venison in a food processor and briefly pulse until it looks like mince. Heat 1 tbsp of the olive oil in a non-stick frying pan and fry the venison on medium heat until it is no longer pink. Set aside.

Heat the remaining olive oil in a frying pan and add all the diced and chopped vegetables, apart from the peas. Fry for several minutes until slightly cooked but still crunchy.

Add the venison (and its juice) to the vegetables. Add the tomato paste, stock cube, rosemary, Worcestershire sauce, cinnamon and 125ml water. Heat through for another minute. Season to taste.

Transfer the vegetable and venison mix to a lightly oiled casserole dish. Sprinkle frozen peas over the top in a single light layer. With a spoon, gently spread the mashed sweet potato over the top.

Bake for 30–40 minutes, until piping hot and slightly browned around the edges.

BEAR'S 30-MINUTE
SUPER-LEAN CHILLI

Serves 4–6

800g grass-fed organic venison, beef or buffalo, cubed

2 tbsp olive oil

1 large onion, skinned and chopped

4 garlic cloves, skinned and finely chopped

2 chillies, very finely chopped

1 red pepper, deseeded and cut into small cubes

1 green pepper, deseeded and cut into small cubes

1 tsp ground coriander

1 tsp dried marjoram

2 tsp paprika

2 tsp dried oregano

½ tsp cinnamon

1½ tsp Worcestershire sauce (or tamari sauce if you want to be gluten-free)

½ tsp cayenne pepper

1 heaped tsp raw cacao powder

4 tbsp tomato paste

1 tsp ground black pepper

2 tins chopped tomatoes

salt, to taste (at least 1 heaped tsp)

400g tin kidney beans (optional)

Super-quick, super-easy and super-lean – with an amazing kick. Great for freezing in big batches or eating throughout the week.

Put the beef, buffalo or venison in a food processor and pulse into a mince.

Heat the olive oil in a large frying pan and fry the onion, garlic and chilli for several minutes. Add the mince and the pepper and fry until the meat is no longer pink, using a fork to break up any large chunks.

Add all the spices, herbs, Worcestershire sauce, cacao powder and tomato paste and bring to a simmer. Simmer for several minutes, then add the chopped tomatoes, salt, and kidney beans if you're using them. Simmer for another 5–10 minutes and your chilli is done. Easy!

Serve with some boiled quinoa, home-made Foolproof Guacamole (see page 202) and a side salad for a complete meal.

MEDITERRANEAN QUICHE

Serves 4

For the crust
90g oats
140g sunflower seeds
1 tsp dried oregano
1 tbsp olive oil
salt to taste (about ¼ tsp)

For the filling
olive oil
2 large garlic cloves,
    skinned and finely
    chopped
1 red onion, skinned
    and finely diced
3 spring onions,
    finely sliced
10 black olives, finely sliced
5 sun-dried tomatoes in oil,
    finely chopped
a handful of fresh basil
    leaves, finely chopped
1 tsp fresh rosemary,
    finely chopped
2 tbsp nutritional
    yeast flakes
400g tofu
salt and pepper

This quiche is free from milk, eggs, cheese, wheat, gluten and nuts. So: suitable for almost anyone! People can't believe how good this tastes with no eggs or cheese.

Preheat the oven to 175°C/350°F/gas mark 4.

To make the crust, blitz the oats and sunflower seeds in a food processor to a flour-like consistency. Mix in the oregano, oil and salt. Use your hands to knead the mixture into a dough.

Lightly oil a 20cm quiche tin and spread out the dough to cover the bottom of the tin, using your fingers to press it down firmly and evenly to the edges. Once the bottom is covered, use a fork to pierce the dough all over. Bake for approximately 15 minutes, or until firm to the touch.

In the meantime, make the filling. Heat some olive oil in a frying pan, then sauté the garlic, onion and spring onions for several minutes until soft. Turn off the heat and add all the other ingredients apart from the tofu.

Take the tofu out of its packet and squeeze it over a bowl with both hands, as firmly as you can, to get as much liquid out of it as possible. Discard the liquid and transfer the squeezed tofu to a food processor. Add 1 tbsp of olive oil and blitz until the tofu has a smooth, creamy consistency. Transfer the creamed tofu to the pan with all the remaining ingredients and stir until everything is well combined.

Spoon the thick mixture on top of your cooked quiche crust and bake in the oven at 190°C/375°F/gas mark 5 for about 30 minutes, or until firm to the touch and slightly browned on top.

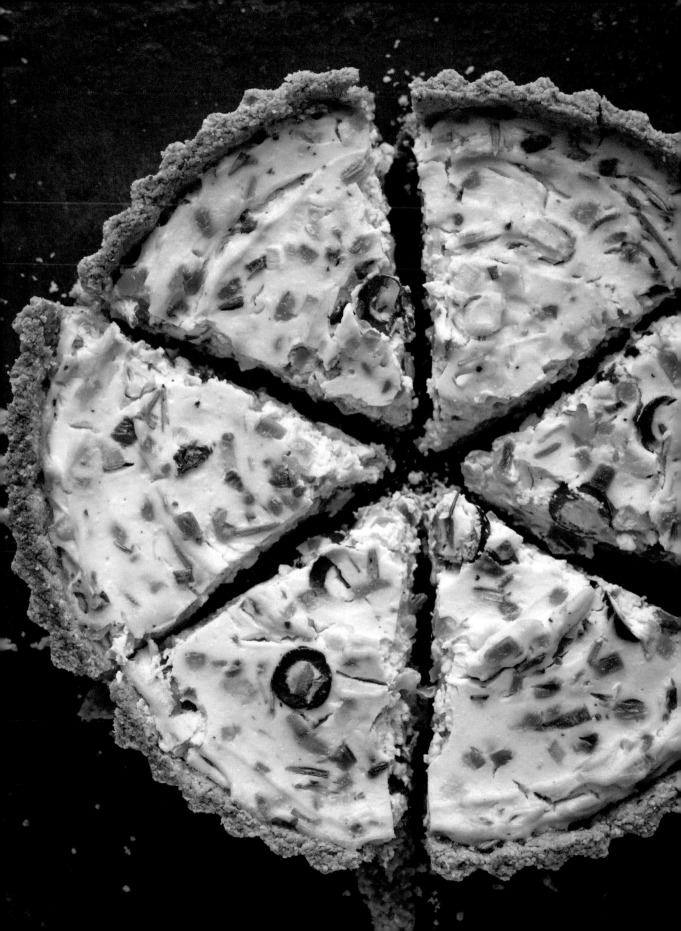

BEAR'S LUXURY
NUT ROAST

Serves 4–6 as a meat replacement for your Sunday roast

3 tbsp finely ground flax seeds (see page 71)

2 garlic cloves, skinned and finely chopped

1 red onion, skinned and finely chopped

1 leek, white part only, finely chopped

1 medium carrot, grated

1 celery stalk, finely chopped

a handful of fresh parsley, finely chopped

1 tsp fresh thyme, chopped

250g mixed nuts (e.g. cashews, Brazils, walnuts or hazelnuts; if you have a nut allergy, use mixed seeds)

90g oats

400g tin butter beans, drained

150ml vegetable stock

salt and pepper

a dash of cayenne pepper (optional)

I don't like the name 'nut roast' as it does always sound very geeky! But actually, this is both delicious and filling, and is perfect for a family veg dish.

Preheat the oven to 180°C/350°F/gas mark 4. Line a loaf tin (approximately 21 x 11 x 7cm) with baking paper and lightly grease it with olive oil.

Mix the ground flax seed in a bowl with 9 tbsp water. Set aside to soak for at least 10 minutes.

In a frying pan, lightly sauté the garlic and onion in a little olive oil. Add the leek, carrot, celery, parsley and thyme. Sauté for a few more minutes. Remove from the heat.

Pulse the nuts in a food processor until they are broken into small pieces. Don't mix for too long – they should not be too fine. Remove from the processor and set aside.

Blitz the oats to a fine powder in your food processor. Add the butter beans and pulse until you have a creamy mixture. Add the soaked flax, vegetable stock, some salt and pepper (approximately ½ tsp salt and 12 grinds of pepper) and pulse again until you have a thick, creamy mixture.

Add the oat and bean mixture to the vegetables, then stir in the chopped nuts. Mix well and check the seasoning (add cayenne pepper if you like).

Transfer the mixture to the loaf tin and bake for about 45 minutes. Remove from the oven and turn the tin over so that the loaf slides out. Place the loaf upside down on a baking tray lined with a new piece of baking paper. Return to the oven for another 20–30 minutes to brown all over.

The loaf tastes lovely and meaty and turns out quite moist. If you want it dryer, divide the mixture between two smaller loaf tins, or leave it in the oven for 5–15 minutes longer.

MEAN BEAN BURGER

Makes 4–6 burgers

1 tin black beans (about 230g, drained and rinsed)

½ small red onion, skinned and very finely chopped

¼ green pepper, deseeded and finely chopped

1–2 garlic cloves, skinned and minced

½ medium carrot, grated

1 tsp chipotle paste

½ tsp cumin

3 tbsp oats

a handful of coriander, finely chopped

½ tsp smoked paprika

1 egg

1 tbsp whole flax seeds

a dash of Worcestershire sauce (leave out if you're vegan, vegetarian or gluten-intolerant)

1 tbsp olive oil, plus extra for greasing

¼ tsp salt

black pepper

NB: use a Flax Egg if you can't have eggs (see page 201).

These burgers are cheap and easy to make. The base recipe of most bean burgers is pretty much the same, using vegetables for moisture and flavour. I've given these a nice spicy kick with chipotle, but you can add any other spices that rock your boat. You could also use kidney beans, lentils or chickpeas instead of black beans, or replace some of the beans with sunflower seeds for a 'heavier' version. These come out looking pretty much like large chocolate chip cookies, and taste good both hot and cold.

Preheat the oven to 180°C/350°F/gas mark 4. Line a baking tray with baking paper, and lightly oil this as well (the patties can stick).

Pulse all the ingredients in a food processor until you have a smooth, thick consistency. Spoon out 2 tbsp mixture per burger on to the baking tray and shape like a burger.

Bake for 15 minutes until set, flip over carefully and bake for another 10–15 minutes until cooked in the centre and crisp on the outside.

These taste great on a Portobello Bun (see page 208), served with some rocket, a large dollop of Foolproof Guacamole (page 202) and some Sweet Potato Chips (page 216).

POWER PIZZA

Makes 1 pizza

For the base

5 tbsp chia seeds
4 heaped tbsp buckwheat
  flour
1 tbsp olive oil
200ml water
1 tbsp fresh rosemary
1 tsp oregano
½ tsp salt

For the sauce

a handful of cherry
  tomatoes (around 12),
  or a 400g tin chopped
  tomatoes, drained
3 heaped tbsp tomato paste
2 garlic cloves, skinned
  and chopped
some fresh rosemary
  or basil, chopped
2 tbsp nutritional
  yeast flakes
a splash of olive or hemp oil
a generous pinch of salt

For the topping

Whatever you fancy! Choose
from: finely sliced red onion;
sun-dried tomatoes; olives;
thinly sliced courgette;
tiny broccoli florets; thinly
sliced mushrooms; thinly
sliced peppers; fresh basil;
a couple of handfuls of
rocket or spinach (add
these only for the last
few minutes of baking); a
generous drizzle of olive oil

This pizza base is wheat- and gluten-free, filling, nutrient-dense and packed with protein, fibre and healthy fats. Real power food.

Preheat the oven to 175°C/350°F/gas mark 4.

Mix together all ingredients for the base using a fork or a whisk until it forms a thick batter and slowly turns into a blob, which will happen as the chia seeds start to soak up the water. If you feel it isn't thick enough, add a little more buckwheat flour – but give it a few minutes to thicken up before doing this.

Line a round, 28cm baking tray with baking paper and lightly oil it with olive oil. Drop the thick batter on to the tray and spread out the mixture evenly with the back of a spoon. It wants to be just under 1cm thick. Bake for about 40–45 minutes.

Meanwhile, blitz all the sauce ingredients until you have a very smooth, thick sauce. (You can add a bit of water or olive oil if it seems too thick.)

Spread the sauce over the baked pizza base, then add your topping of choice, drizzle with a little olive oil and bake for another 5–10 minutes until the veggies are cooked through.

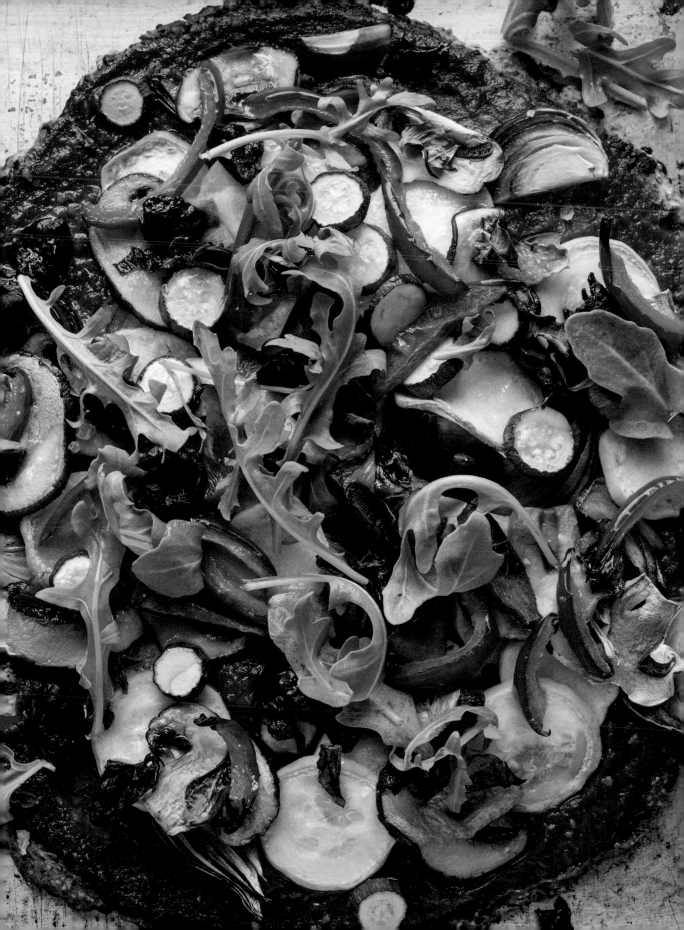

BEAR'S BUFFALO BURGER

Makes 4 burgers

500g ground buffalo meat

1 tbsp tomato paste

½ small red onion, skinned and finely chopped

1–2 garlic cloves, skinned and finely chopped

several generous dashes of Worcestershire sauce (don't use if you're vegetarian, vegan or gluten-free)

salt and pepper, to taste

A burger doesn't have to be junk food: it can be super-nutritious, depending on how it's prepared and what it's served with. I've gone off buying cheap minced meat altogether. If I have a burger, I like it to be real meat. I love buffalo: it's naturally much lower in fat than beef, but still tender and with none of the added nasties such as hormones or antibiotics. You can get it from specialist butchers and farms throughout the UK.

Mix all the ingredients together in a bowl. Don't overwork it – buffalo meat doesn't need a lot of tampering with.

Form into four burgers. It's best to stick them in the fridge for an hour, but you can cook them straight away.

Heat a little olive oil in a frying pan and fry for approximately 5 minutes on each side, or until medium-rare – you really don't want to overcook buffalo meat or it will go dry. Alternatively, cook them under a hot grill, turning halfway through, until medium-rare.

Serve on a Portobello Bun (page 208) with a rainbow salad and some Bear-style Fried Sweet Potatoes (page 216)

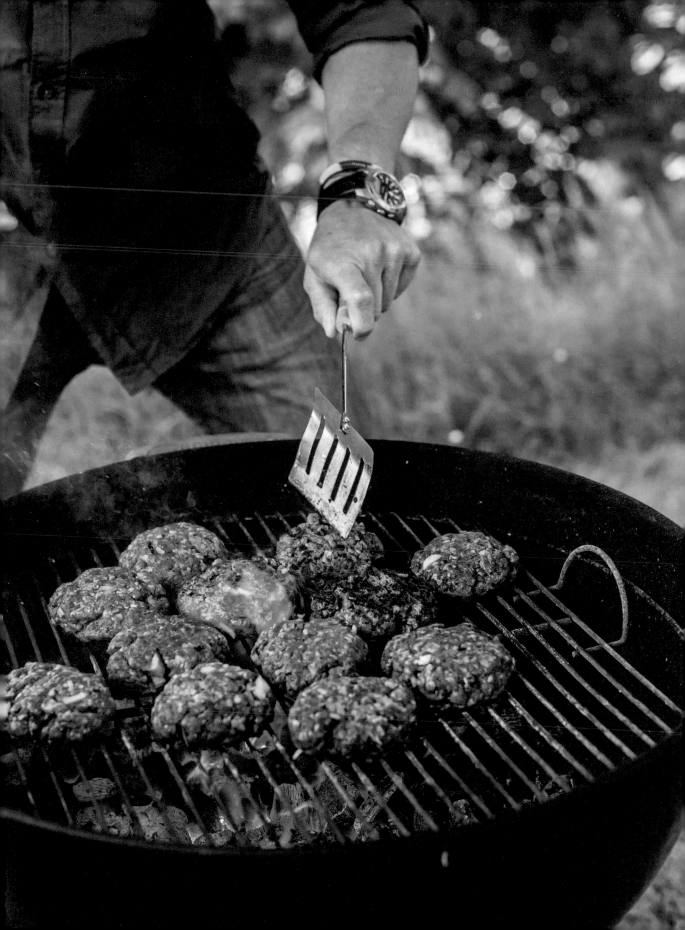

BEAR'S FAVOURITE
THAI CURRY

Serves 4

For the curry paste

3 red or green chillies (less if
you don't like things too hot)

6 garlic cloves, skinned

2 stalks fresh or dried
lemongrass or the equivalent
in lemongrass paste

4cm piece of ginger, peeled
(use galangal instead of
ginger if you can get it)

juice of 1 lime

2 tsp crushed kaffir lime leaves,
or the grated rind of ½ lime

2 shallots, finely sliced

1 small red onion, skinned
and finely diced

2 tsp fish sauce, or 1½ tbsp tamari
sauce if you're vegetarian

6 coriander stalks, finely chopped
(don't throw away the leaves!)

a pinch of cumin powder

1–2 tbsp coconut oil for frying

pepper, to taste

For the vegetables

200g broccoli florets

200g sweet potato, peeled
and cubed

200g aubergine, cubed

4–6 mushrooms, sliced

200g mangetout, green beans
or sugar snap peas

400ml tin coconut milk

½ stock cube

1 tsp coconut palm sugar

a small bunch of coriander,
leaves freshly chopped

Although ready-made curry sauces can appear tempting, they are often just full of sugar and bad fats. Don't be daunted by the idea of making your own. It really isn't that hard and nothing beats the satisfaction, aromas and health benefits of making a curry from scratch. Here's my favourite recipe. You don't have to be too precise with the vegetable measurements or types, though. Just throw in whatever you fancy, so long as it has nice colours and includes something green like broccoli.

Put all the paste ingredients except the coconut oil in a blender or food processor and blend to a paste.

Melt the coconut oil in a pan on medium heat and sauté the paste for a minute or two to extract the flavours from the spices. (Don't let it burn.)

Add the vegetables (apart from the chopped coriander) and the coconut milk. Fill the empty coconut milk tin with water and add some of this – how much depends on how thick you want your curry to be. Let this simmer for several minutes. Add the stock powder and palm sugar and continue simmering until the vegetables are tender.

Serve in a bowl with some brown rice and sprinkle some fresh coriander on top.

For a bit of extra protein, you could add some diced tofu, tempeh, chicken or prawns when you're frying the curry paste. Or add a tin of chickpeas several minutes before the vegetables are done.

If you make double portions of the curry paste, you can freeze it to use again: it will keep for several weeks.

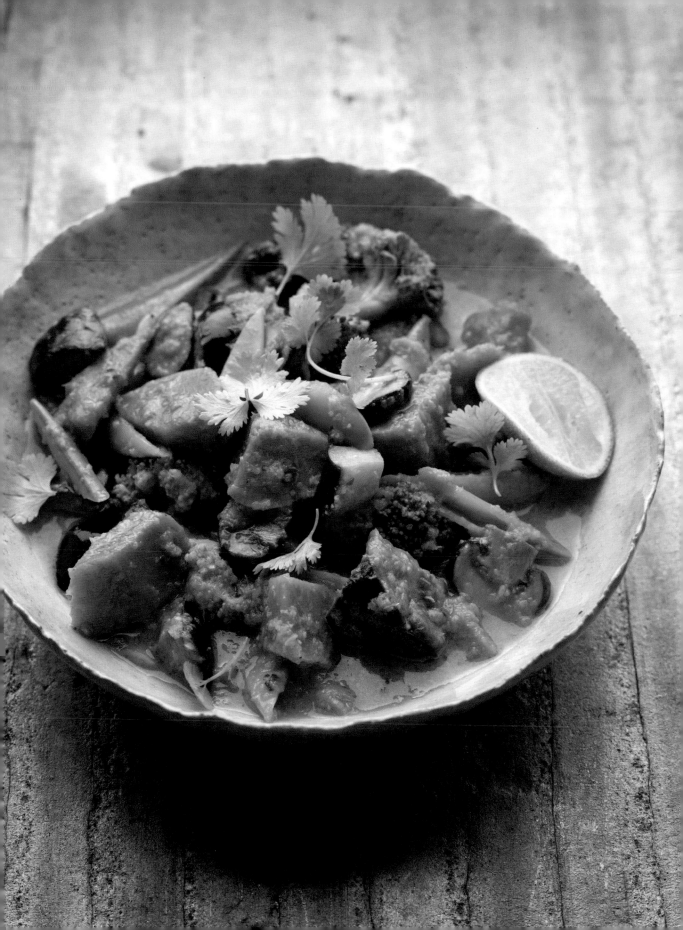

STIR-FRIES

Per person

Approx. 300g chopped, diced or sliced vegetables vegetables that work well in a stir-fry are: green beans, kale, cabbage, beansprouts, peppers, mushrooms, spring onion, grated carrot, grated courgette, sugar snap peas, mangetout, spring greens, Savoy cabbage, small broccoli or cauliflower florets, tenderstem broccoli, asparagus, bok choi, green peas, onion (any kind), spinach (add this at the end), sweet potato.

You can also choose from the following protein sources per person:
80–100g chicken, fish or prawns
100g tofu or tempeh
150g cooked beans or pulses
2 small handfuls of nuts, such as cashew nuts
2 eggs

I love stir-fries. They are quite possibly the easiest, tastiest way to get in a load of different vegetables and a good portion of lean protein. You can have a different-flavoured stir-fry each day of the week and whip it up in about 10 minutes. So if you don't fancy cooking something unknown but still want something new, stir-fries are the way forward. Use whatever leftover veg, herbs and spices you have in your fridge and cupboard to create Thai, Indian, Japanese, Chinese or Italian flavours – or be bold and mix them all together! Here are some guidelines.

I usually start all my Asian-style stir-fries by frying a chopped onion (red or white), a few cloves of garlic, 2.5cm finely chopped ginger and a chopped chilli in 1 tbsp coconut oil. I then add my flavour of choice and protein of choice if it needs cooking (meat, fish, tofu or tempeh) and stir-fry on a medium heat until the protein is almost done (takes about 5 minutes). Then I add my vegetables and stir-fry on a high heat until they're *al dente*. Several minutes before finishing I add any beans, pulses or nuts I might be using. (Don't add them at the very end, as they need to soak up the flavour a bit.)

If I fancy a 'wet' stir-fry, I add ½ tin coconut milk (about 200ml) with the vegetables, and sometimes a little vegetable stock. And if I have any leftover quinoa or brown rice, I serve it on the side or add it to the wok towards the end.

Double or quadruple all the amounts, depending on how many people you're cooking for.

When it comes to sauces, I sometimes use small amounts of pre-made curry pastes to give my stir-fry a different flavour. But if you want to cook fresh, give the following a go:

Thai: Use the curry paste recipe on page 150.

Indian: On a medium heat, fry the following in a little oil with some chopped onion and garlic: a cube freshly chopped ginger, 1 tsp cumin seeds, 1–2 tsp garam masala, 1 tsp nigella seeds, 1 tsp chilli powder. Then add your vegetables and protein. This works best with cauliflower florets, sliced onions, peppers, sliced cabbage and grated carrot.

Italian: Vegetables that work well include courgettes, broccoli, plenty of plum tomatoes, onions and mushrooms. Then chop in some fresh herbs: basil, thyme and dried oregano. Use organic, free-range chicken for protein. Use olive oil for frying. Serve with a portion of buckwheat or brown-rice spaghetti, available at health shops.

Japanese: Make a sauce from 2 tsp finely chopped ginger, 2–4 tbsp sesame oil, 2 tbsp tamari sauce or soy sauce, 2 tbsp rice vinegar, 1–2 tbsp palm sugar or maple syrup. Vegetables that work well with this are: peppers, broccoli, garlic, shitake mushrooms, thinly sliced cabbage. Use grass-fed beef cut into small chunks for protein.

If you're lost for flavours, just add a few tablespoons of hummus and some freshly squeezed lemon to your stir-fried vegetables.

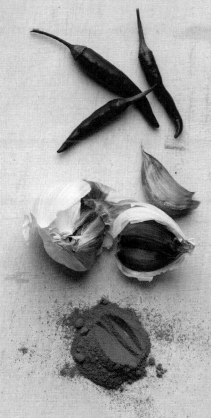

FISH PARCELS
FROM THE OVEN (OR CAMPFIRE!)

Serves 4

4 fish fillets – any fish
   is good
2.5cm piece of ginger,
   peeled and finely chopped
4 garlic cloves, skinned
   and finely chopped
1 medium red chilli, seeded
   and finely chopped
juice of a large lime
   (or more if you like
   it extra zesty)
4–6 tbsp tamari sauce
   or soy sauce
200g mangetout
200g tenderstem broccoli

This is the easiest way there is to cook fish. Just let the oven and the steam inside the parcels do the job for you. You can make the parcels as big or small as you like, using different types of vegetables or fish.

Preheat the oven to 180°C/350°F/gas mark 4.

To make four individual fish parcels, lay each fillet on a piece of tin foil. Evenly spread the ginger, garlic, chilli and lime juice over the fillets. Lay the broccoli and mangetout evenly over the fish, then pour the tamari or soy sauce over the vegetables.

Now gather up the edges of the foil and seal them together to make a package. The fish and vegetables will steam in their own juices, so make sure there is enough 'steaming' space at the top of your parcel. The foil should be tightly closed with no gaps.

Put the fish parcels in a baking tin and cook in the oven for 15–25 minutes. The timing may need adjusting slightly, depending on the thickness and the type of fish you use. Check if it is done after approximately 15 minutes. If not, re-close the package and steam for another 5 minutes, or until cooked through.

Serve with stir-fried vegetables and a small portion of brown basmati rice or wild rice.

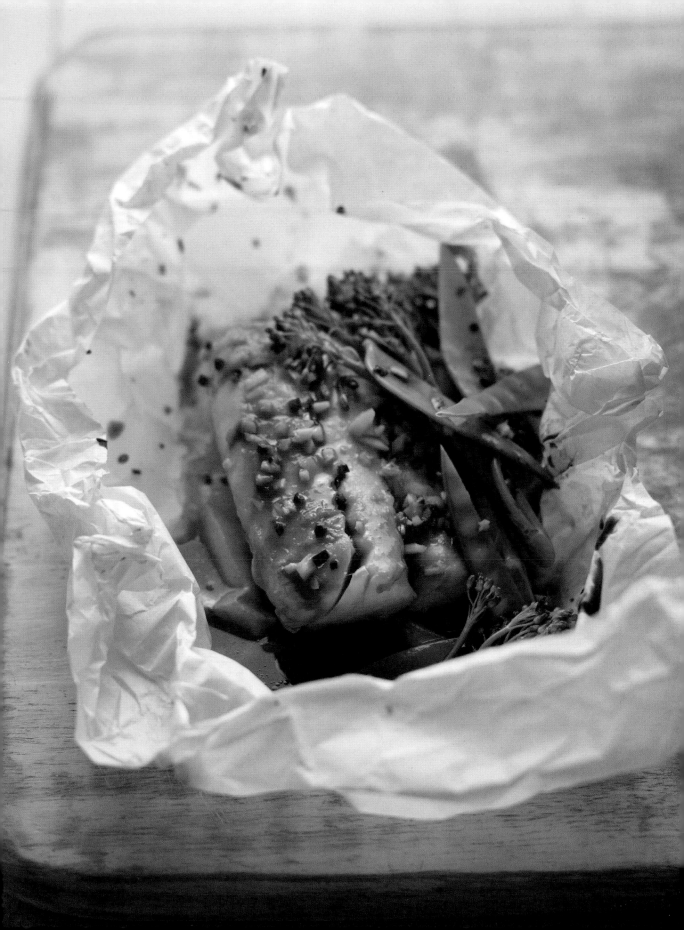

CASHEW LASAGNE

Enough for 2 large portions (for 4, double both the quantities and the size of the dish)

For the white sauce

150g cashews, soaked for a minimum of 2 hours
100ml water
1½ tbsp lemon
2 tbsp nutritional yeast
2 eggs
a dash of nutmeg
½ tsp salt
freshly ground black pepper

For the tomato sauce

400g tin tomatoes (or 2–3 large beef tomatoes)
4–6 garlic cloves, skinned and chopped
4 tbsp tomato paste
2 tbsp olive oil
2 tbsp mixed herbs
a large handful of fresh basil
salt, to taste (approx. ½ tsp)

For the filling

½ large courgette
½ large aubergine
5 large chestnut mushrooms
about 50g spinach leaves

This lasagne is a great source of protein, even though there's no milk, cheese, wheat or meat in it. The cashews need to be soaked for a few hours, so stick them in some water before you leave for work – they'll be ready to use when you start cooking in the evening.

Preheat the oven to 190°C/375°F/gas mark 5.

Drain your soaked cashews. Blend them with the 100ml of water and the lemon juice in a food processor until you have an almost smooth mixture. Keep blending and scraping the sides to make sure all the cashews get blitzed – the end result will be smooth but very slightly grainy. Add the remaining white sauce ingredients and blitz again. Transfer to a bowl.

Put all the tomato sauce ingredients in a blender or food processor and mix until you have a smooth sauce. Slice the courgettes, aubergines and mushrooms very finely.

Grease a 24 x 24cm baking dish with olive oil and layer the bottom with the finely sliced courgettes. The slices don't need to overlap much. Slice a bit more courgette if it doesn't cover the entire base. Pour a third of the tomato sauce on top of this and spread it out evenly. Now lay the sliced mushrooms on top in the same manner. Cover with a third of the white sauce and a little bit of the tomato sauce, spreading the two sauces evenly on top of each other. Layer the sliced aubergine evenly on top, then add another layer of tomato sauce. It doesn't need to be very thick, so don't feel you have to use it all. Arrange the spinach leaves on top in a fine layer and cover with the remaining white sauce, evenly spread.

Cover your tray with aluminium foil and bake for about 40 minutes, or until set and slightly browned around the edges.

COURGETTE AND CARROT SPAGHETTI
WITH AVOCADO PESTO

Per person

1 medium courgette

1 medium carrot, peeled

a handful of basil

½ large, ripe avocado

1 tbsp lemon juice

1 garlic clove, skinned

2 tbsp olive oil and a little
extra for frying

a small handful of pine nuts
or sunflower seeds

cherry tomatoes (optional)

salt and pepper

Courgette pasta has become increasingly popular in the past few years. It's definitely a staple in my house. You can make it the fancy way with a spiralizer or mandoline, or do what I do and use a plain old box-grater or a peeler.

To make the spaghetti, put a box-grater on its side with the thickest grater facing up, then move your courgette and carrot lengthwise along it to create long strips. Or simply use a peeler to create thin slices.

Heat a little olive oil in a pan and sauté the courgette and carrot slices for several minutes until softened. Grind a little black pepper over the top. Set aside.

In a blender, blitz all the remaining ingredients, apart from the pine nuts or sunflower seeds and the tomatoes, to a smooth, creamy sauce.

Briefly roast the pine nuts in a dry pan until golden brown (no need to do this if you're using sunflower seeds).

Mix the sauce with the spaghetti and sprinkle the pine nuts on top. If you like, add some (grilled) diced cherry tomatoes.

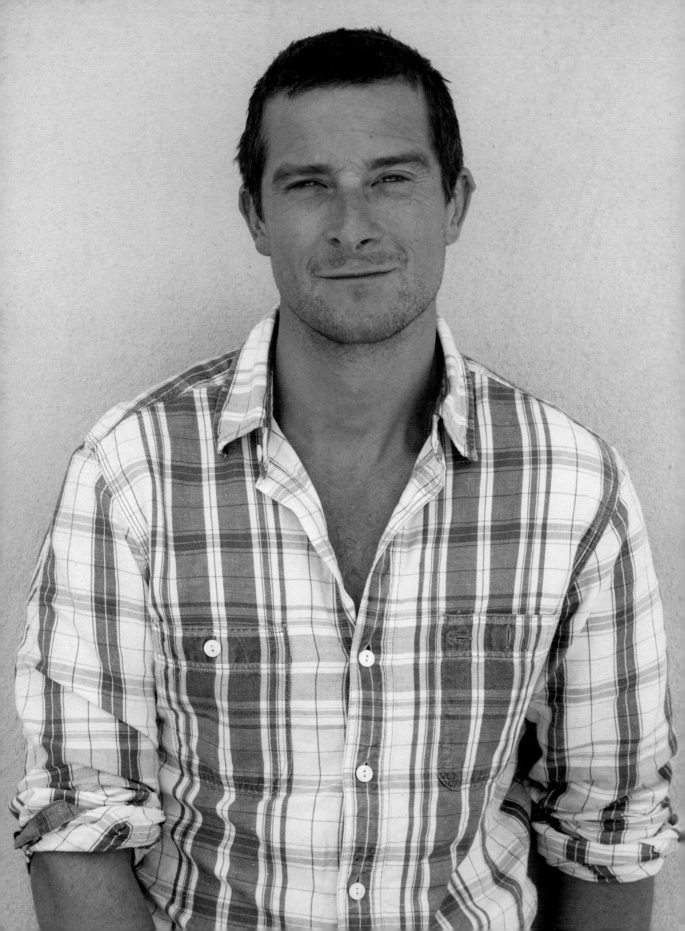

FILLING MEALTIME SOUPS & HOTPOTS

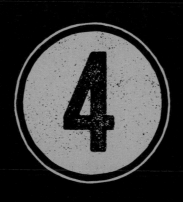

You know the feeling: it's cold and wet outside, and it seems to drain you of energy. These recipes are the answer. They'll keep you fuelled and full, yet also help to keep you trim. They provide a bulk of nutrients in one bowl and I eat meals like this several times a week. You can cook all these in big batches and freeze them for the weeks ahead.

IMMUNE-BOOSTING
AUTUMN SOUP

Serves 2

1 onion, skinned
   and chopped
2 garlic cloves, skinned
   and chopped
2 carrots, chopped
600ml vegetable stock
100g shitake mushrooms
150g chestnut mushrooms
200g vacuum-packed
   cooked chestnuts
black pepper, to taste

This soup tastes super-creamy without the use of cream. Serve it as a starter to a light meal, or have it as a main meal in a large bowl served with some Healthy Herby Bread (page 205).

Put the chopped onion, garlic and carrots in a large pot, pour in the stock, bring to the boil, then simmer for 15 minutes.

Add the mushrooms and chestnuts and simmer for a further 10 minutes. Season to taste with black pepper.

Use a food processor or hand blender to purée the soup till you have a smooth, creamy mixture.

CHARGE-YOUR-MUSCLES
BEETROOT SOUP

Serves 2

2 medium beetroots

1 tbsp olive or coconut oil

1 onion, skinned and
    chopped

2 garlic cloves, skinned
    and chopped

1 tsp chopped ginger

2 stalks celery, finely diced

600ml vegetable stock

a pinch of cumin

½ tsp English mustard

sea salt and black pepper

3 tbsp coconut cream,
    oat cream or soya cream
    (optional)

Beetroot helps to oxygenate the muscles and can enhance performance when exercising. Serve with some Herby Bread (page 205) to charge yourself for your evening workout.

Boil the fresh beetroots with their skin on for 30–45 minutes, until soft enough to pierce with a sharp knife. Cut off the ends and chop into pieces.

Heat the oil in a large pot and sauté the onion, garlic and ginger for 2 minutes. Add the beetroot, celery and vegetable stock. Bring to the boil and simmer until the beetroot has softened enough to blend.

Put in a blender with the cumin, mustard, salt and pepper. Blend until smooth. Add the coconut, soya or oat cream to make the soup even creamier.

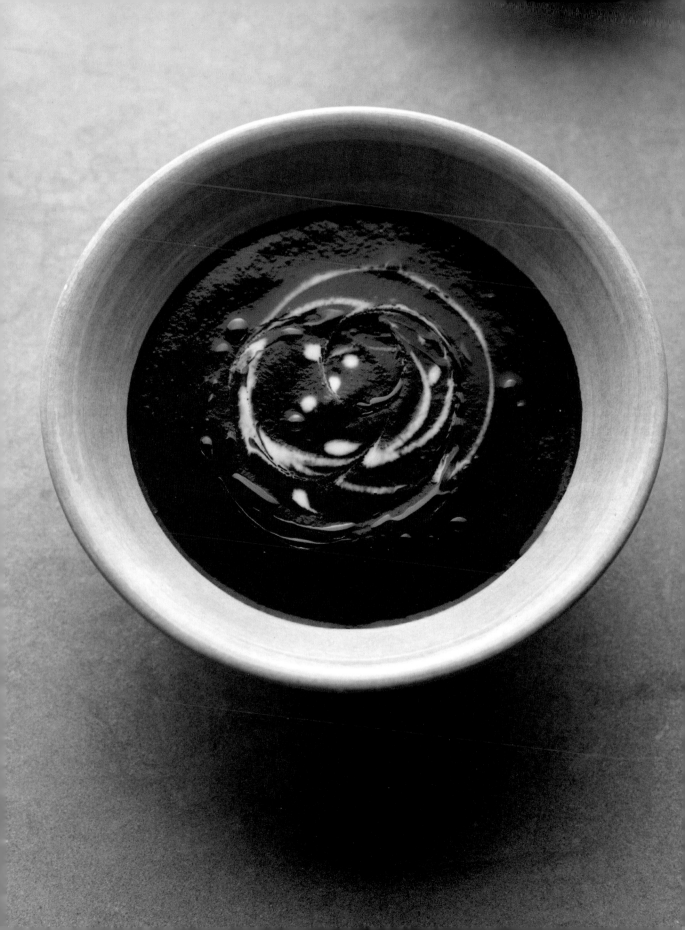

CLEAN-UP-YOUR-ACT
SOUP

Serves 4

1 tbsp olive or coconut oil

2 garlic cloves, skinned and chopped

1 onion, skinned and finely chopped

2.5cm piece of fresh ginger, peeled and finely chopped

1 head fresh broccoli (400–500g), cut into small florets

2 medium parsnips, peeled and chopped

2 stalks celery, finely chopped

100g spinach leaves

juice of ½ small lemon

sea salt and ground pepper, to taste

This soup is super-clean, super-green and zesty. Everything you need to help your body get rid of excess toxins. It's filling on its own, no bread needed. Great to detox the body.

In a large pot, heat the oil and stir in the garlic, onion and ginger. Sauté for 1–2 minutes until soft, then add the broccoli, parsnips and celery.

Add water: 250ml for a thick soup, 500ml for a thinner one. Bring to the boil, then reduce to a simmer. Now put the spinach on top and cover the pot. Cook until all the veggies are softened.

Use a blender or food processor to purée the soup. Once blended, add the lemon juice, then season with salt and pepper.

To make this soup creamier, add a dash of coconut milk when serving.

SPICY BUTTERNUT SQUASH SOUP

Serves 2

1 garlic clove, skinned and finely chopped

1 medium onion, skinned and finely chopped

1 tbsp coconut oil

600g butternut squash, peeled and cubed

150ml vegetable stock

¾ tsp curry powder

½ tin (80ml) coconut cream (to taste)

a dash of Worcestershire sauce

freshly ground pepper and sea salt

½ tbsp pumpkin seeds per person

This is Kay's favourite soup. One bowl never seems to be enough. Warming, nourishing, filling – great for a cold winter's day.

Melt the coconut oil in a pot on medium heat and fry the onion and garlic until softened. Add the butternut squash cubes and stir for 1 more minute.

Add the vegetable stock and curry powder, then simmer until the squash is soft (approximately 20–25 minutes).

Pour in the coconut cream and then, with a potato masher, mash the ingredients to a soup consistency. Season to taste with Worcestershire sauce, salt and pepper. Pour into bowls and sprinkle pumpkin seeds on top.

STAMINA STEW

Serves 4–6

olive oil for frying
1 large onion, skinned
   and finely chopped
4 garlic cloves, skinned
   and finely chopped
1 red pepper, finely diced
200g kale, thick stems
   removed and leaves
   finely chopped
8 cherry tomatoes,
   finely diced
300g quinoa
4 tbsp lemon juice
400g tin chickpeas, drained
2 tbsp nutritional yeast
600ml hot vegetable stock
100ml soya or oat cream
2 tsp dried oregano
1 tsp freshly ground pepper
salt, to taste (at least
   ½ tsp)
a dash of cayenne pepper

Kale is one of the healthiest vegetables in the world, and quinoa is one of the healthiest pseudo grains. Put them together, you've got a real health kick! This casserole is full of protein, fibre, calcium, magnesium, vitamins – and flavour. Great for a light lunch or served as a side to venison steak . . .

Preheat the oven to 220°C/425°F/gas mark 7.

Heat a little olive oil in a frying pan and fry the onion, garlic and red pepper for several minutes. Add the chopped kale and chopped tomatoes, and continue to fry on a low heat for a few more minutes until the kale has softened up.

Rinse the quinoa and transfer to a casserole. Add the kale mix and all the remaining ingredients. Stir until everything is well combined.

Cover the casserole with tin foil and put it in the oven. Check after 20 minutes to see if all the liquid has been absorbed. If not, bake for a further 5–10 minutes.

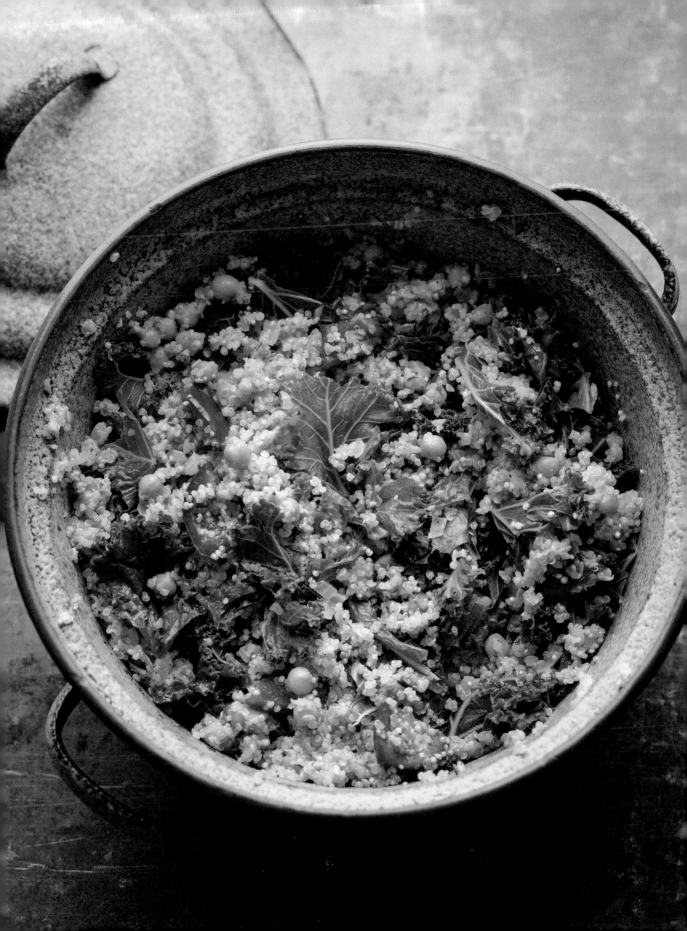

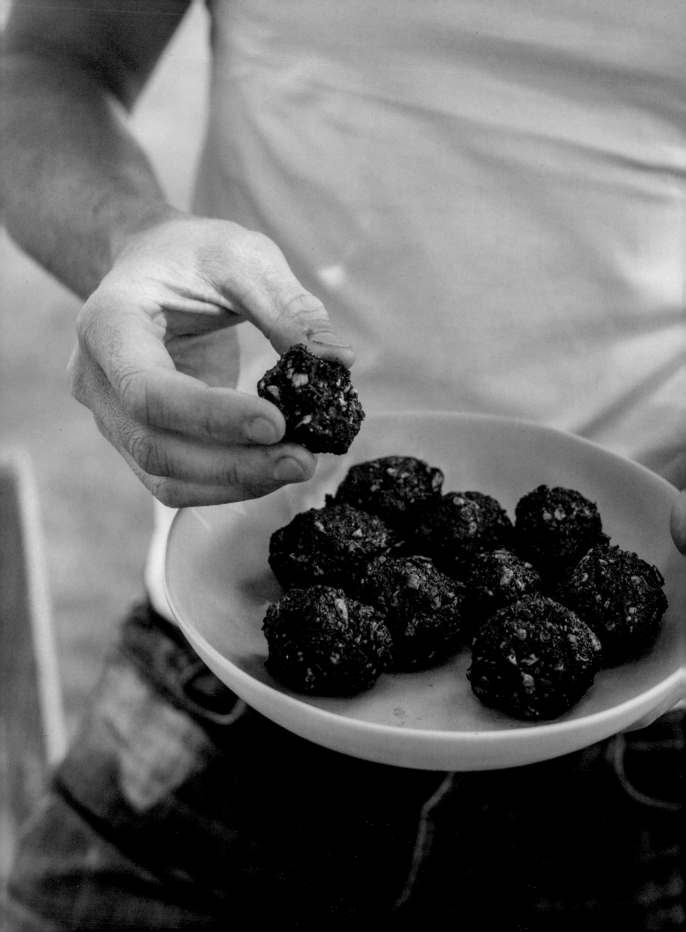

SNACKS

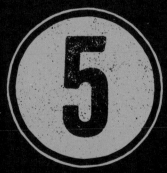

Snacks keep me going when I'm out and about – not just when I'm on the trail, but in everyday life, which is always busy – so I've become kind of dependent on them. It was a challenge for me to find snacks that fuelled me properly and tasted great, but which were also mega-healthy. This selection provides you with exactly that: super-healthy, super-tasty pick-me-ups for the middle of a hectic day, or a much-needed energy boost pre- or post-workout.

PROTEIN BOMBS

Makes about 10

2 heaped tbsp coconut oil
50g hemp protein powder
40g raw cacao powder
75g sunflower seeds
1 tbsp virgin olive oil (not
    the strong-tasting kind)
a pinch of salt
½ tsp stevia powder
125g dates
4 tbsp water

These filling bombs taste just like the inside of a Mars bar and give you an amazing energy boost. They are my absolute favourite sweet snack. Period. Often to be found in a sandwich bag jammed into my backpack or pockets! But they are definitely best kept cold.

Put the coconut oil in a pan and set over medium heat until it melts.

Place the melted oil in a food processor with the remaining ingredients. Blend until you have a very fine, semi-dry mixture.

Now add water. Start with 4 tbsp and blend again. If it doesn't form into a dough, add a bit more water (1 tbsp at a time) until the mixture turns into a sticky ball.

Now roll the dough into around 10 smaller balls and eat. Or, if you are patient enough, put the dough in the fridge for about 30 minutes before rolling it out, which makes the job easier and less sticky.

NUT BOMBS

Makes about 10

150g mixed nuts
40g raw cacao powder
50g hemp protein powder
xylitol, stevia or maple
    syrup, to taste
desiccated coconut
    (optional)

These are a simpler version of the Protein Bombs on page 171 – fewer ingredients, but just as tasty and just as good for when you are on the go and need that quick energy boost.

Blitz all the ingredients in a food processor with 1–2 tbsp water until they form a ball. Don't add too much water or the mixture will become sticky.

Roll the dough into bite-size balls. If you like, roll each ball through desiccated coconut.

These are ready to eat immediately. Keep in the fridge.

SUPER-QUICK
FIG AND PECAN
ENERGY BARS

Makes about 6

150g figs
100g pecans (or walnuts)
1 tbsp cashew butter

How simple can a snack be? Chewy and sweet, these energy bars are a great post-workout snack.

Mix everything together in a food processor with 2 tbsp water until you have a big ball.

Put the dough into a lightly oiled baking tin, any size. Spread the mixture out and press down gently and evenly with the back of a spoon. Press them down as thick or thin as you like.

Put in the fridge or freezer and allow to set, before cutting into bars.

INSTANT-ENERGY
FLAPJACKS

Makes 10–12

200g pitted dates, chopped
(don't buy pre-chopped
dates – they are too dry
and don't easily form
a paste)
100g coconut oil
100g organic crunchy
peanut butter (no added
sugar or salt)
4 tbsp ground flax seeds
(see page 71)
1 medium-ripe banana,
sliced into tiny pieces
200g oats
1 tsp vanilla extract
a pinch of salt

The awesome, energy-giving trio of peanuts, oats and bananas means that these flapjacks will give you a real kick. These are very popular with our three boys as a snack on the way back from school, to stop them getting tired and grumpy! And with me!

Put the dates in a pan with 100ml water. Set it over low heat and push the dates against the sides of the pan with the back of a spoon so that they mix with the water and become a smooth paste. Add the coconut oil and stir until melted.

Turn off the heat, add the peanut butter and stir until melted. Gently stir in the flax seeds and banana. Add the oats, vanilla extract and salt. Stir until properly mixed.

Transfer the mixture to a lightly oiled square brownie tin (approximately 24 x 24cm), spread it out and press it down gently and evenly with the back of a spoon. (If your tin is bigger or smaller than this, your flapjacks will simply be thicker or thinner – don't worry about it.)

Put in the fridge and allow to set for 30–60 minutes, until you can slice the mixture into small squares. (Although to be honest, it tastes awesome even before it sets!)

ALTERNATIVE: You can replace peanut butter with almond or cashew butter and flax seeds with chia seeds.

SEED BARS

Makes 10–15
200g dates
100g coconut oil
150g mixed seeds (e.g. 50g
   flax, 50g pumpkin, 50g
   sunflower)
150g oats
1 tsp cinnamon
a pinch of salt
desiccated coconut
   (optional)

These are brilliant if you don't have time to make breakfast or if you need instant energy when you're on the trail. I often take these with me when travelling. Also great for kids to take into school, as they contain no nuts.

Put the dates in a pan with 150ml water, and set it over a low heat. Push the dates against the sides of the pan with the back of a spoon so they mix with the water and become a smooth paste. Add the coconut oil and stir until melted.

Turn off the heat. Add the seeds and mix well. Add the oats, cinnamon and salt, and stir everything around until thoroughly mixed.

Transfer the mixture to a lightly oiled square brownie tin (approximately 24 x 24cm), spread it out and press it down gently and evenly with the back of a spoon. (If your tin is bigger or smaller, your seed bars will simply be thicker or thinner – don't worry about it.) If you like, sprinkle some desiccated coconut over the top. With the blunt side of a knife, cut it into squares.

You can either let these set in the fridge for 30–60 minutes and eat them raw (this is how I prefer them), or you can bake them at 180°C/350°F/gas mark 4 for 15 minutes until golden brown (this is how my kids like them).

KALE CHIPS

Serves 2

1 bag (about 200g) kale
1–2 tbsp olive oil
¼ tsp sea salt, more
    or less to taste

Optional flavourings

nutritional yeast flakes
garlic powder
curry powder
black pepper

A great way to get some green leafy vegetables in. People just love these when they come round to my home. The best guilt-free snack out there!

Preheat the oven to 130°C/260°F/gas mark ¾. Line a large baking tray with baking paper.

If you've washed the kale, make sure it is very, very dry. Place it in a large bowl, then add the oil, salt and any optional flavourings you like. Mix quickly with your hands, so that every single leaf has a coating of some oil. (Don't massage for too long, though, or your kale will go limp!)

Lay the kale in a single layer on the prepared baking tray and bake for 8–12 minutes, until just crisp but not brown. (Depending on your oven, the time may need adjusting, but make sure to start checking after 8 minutes that the kale isn't burning.) Serve immediately.

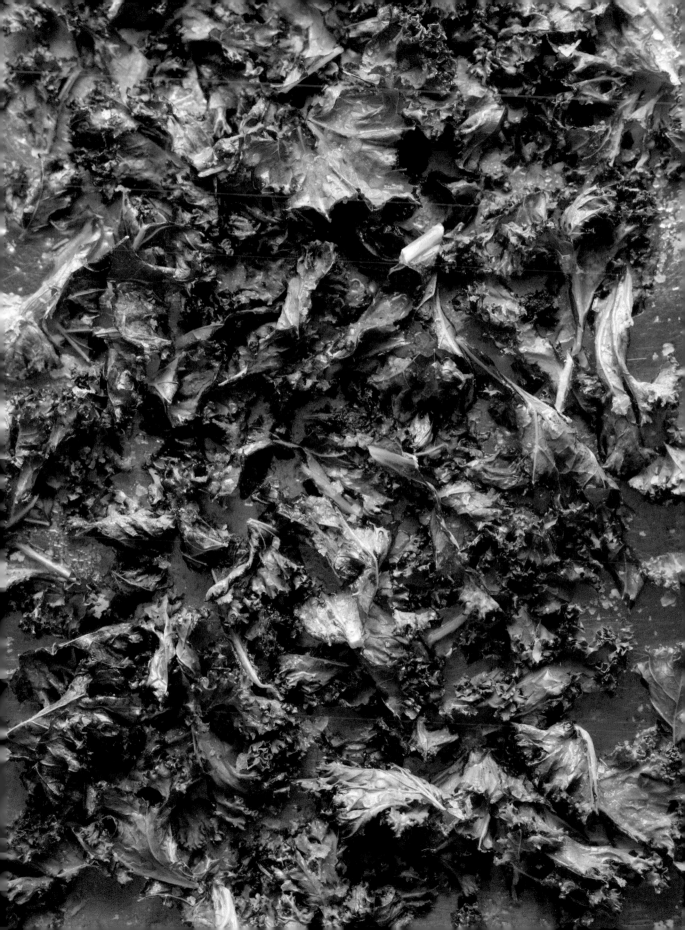

INDIAN QUINOA BITES

Makes 8–10

2 normal eggs or 2 flax eggs
  (see page 201)
1 medium white onion,
  skinned and finely
  chopped
1 large garlic clove, skinned
  and finely chopped
1 small hot chilli (less or
  more, depending how
  spicy you like things)
1 tbsp coconut oil, plus a
  little extra for greasing
½ tsp cumin seeds
½ tsp turmeric powder
2 tsp garam masala
200g sweet potato,
  finely diced
150g quinoa
450ml vegetable stock
150g frozen peas
salt and lots of freshly
  ground pepper

These are great little snacks. They remind me a bit of the Indian samosas we used to eat when I was once climbing in Sikkim. Tasty, filling, healthy.

If using flax eggs, start by making these – see page 201.

Next, melt the coconut oil in a pan on medium heat and fry the onion, garlic and chilli. After 2 minutes add the cumin seeds, turmeric and garam masala, and fry for another minute or two (don't let the spices burn!).

Add the quinoa, sweet potato and the vegetable stock, and boil on a low heat with the lid on for approximately 15 minutes, stirring occasionally, then for 5 minutes with the lid off until the quinoa is as good as done and has a thick, porridge-like consistency.

Take off the heat, leave to cool for 5 minutes and then season with salt and pepper (approximately ½ tsp salt and 12 grinds of pepper). While the quinoa cools down, preheat your oven to 180°C/350°F/gas mark 4 and place paper cases inside the muffin-tin holes. Now add the frozen peas and finally the flax eggs or normal eggs to your quinoa mixture. Mix well.

Put about 2 tbsp of the mixture into each muffin case, then flatten it down with the back of a spoon. Bake the bites for 25–30 minutes until golden brown on top. Leave to cool completely so the bites can set.

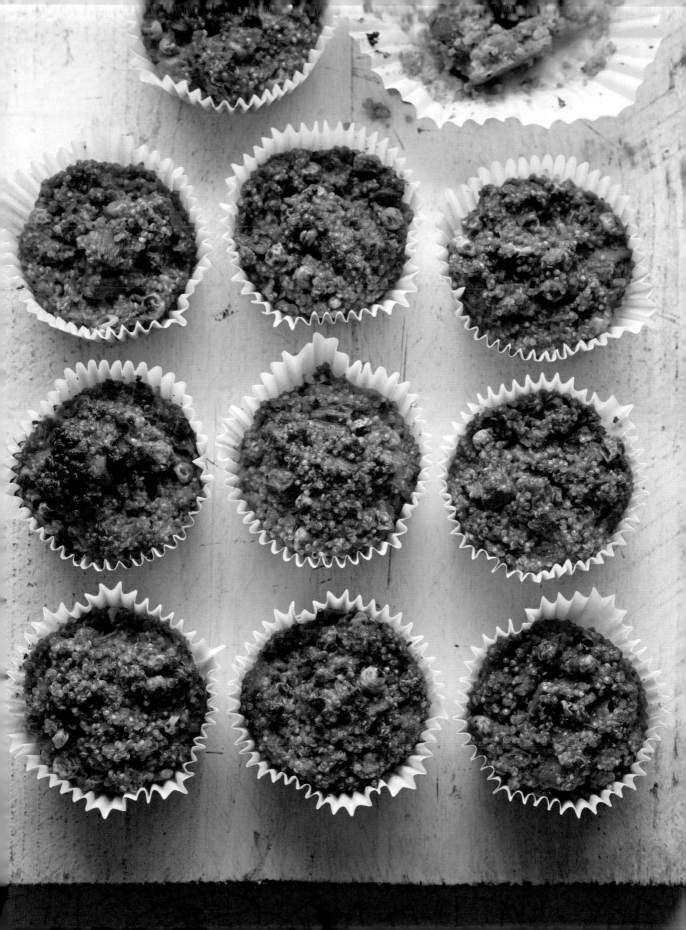

NATURE'S HORLICKS

Per person

1 large cup almond
   or coconut milk
¼ tsp ginger powder
¼ tsp cinnamon
freshly ground black pepper
   (about 3 grindings)
3 cardamom pods, slightly
   crushed
2 dried cloves
a pinch of nutmeg
stevia, to sweeten

This recipe helps to curb the cravings for coffee as well as sweets. Great for digestion and for warming up your body when you just feel like getting cosy.

Put the milk and all the spices in a pan and bring to the boil. Simmer gently for 1 minute, then pour into a large mug. Sweeten to taste with stevia. Drink!

BANANA WALNUT BREAD

Makes 1 loaf

2 heaped tbsp coconut oil

4 ripe medium bananas

100g almond butter

3 large eggs

200g walnut pieces

65g coconut flour (replace with almond flour if you can't find coconut flour, but the taste and consistency will be slightly different)

1 tbsp maple syrup

1 tbsp cinnamon

1 tsp baking powder

1 tsp baking soda

1 tsp vanilla extract

a pinch of salt

As a kid I used to love banana bread more than anything else out there! This recipe rekindles all those positive childhood memories. Best served gooey!

Preheat the oven to 175°C/350°F/gas mark 4. Lightly grease a loaf tin (approximately 21 x 11 x 7cm), then line it with lightly greased baking paper.

Put the coconut oil in a pan and melt over medium heat. Set aside.

Mix the bananas, almond butter and eggs in a food processor (or use a hand blender). Add the melted coconut oil and mix until smooth. Add all remaining ingredients and mix again until properly combined.

Pour the mixture into the loaf tin and bake for 50–60 minutes, or until a toothpick inserted in the centre comes out clean. Don't over-bake or the bread may become dry. Leave in the tin for a few minutes, then turn out on to a wire rack to cool.

COCONUT APRICOT BALLS

Makes 15

150g apricots
100g cashews
½ tsp cinnamon
2 tbsp coconut milk
    (optional)
desiccated coconut,
    to coat

Apricots are nutrient-dense and a great source of dietary fibre, potassium, iron and antioxidants. Great for heart health, digestion and energy. The cashews add proteins and healthy fats. A perfectly balanced snack.

The addition of coconut milk to this recipe helps the other ingredients to bind together and makes the balls slightly creamier, but the recipe works perfectly well without it.

Put all the ingredients apart from the desiccated coconut in a food processor and blitz until the mixture forms a sticky ball.

Using your fingers, make small balls and roll them in desiccated coconut to coat them completely. Done. Keep these in the fridge.

LAYERED CARROT CAKE

Makes 1 cake

For the icing
150g macadamia nuts
2 tbsp lemon juice
2 tbsp coconut oil
75ml maple syrup

For the cake
2 large carrots, peeled and
    chopped into small pieces
130g almond flour
250g dates
40g desiccated coconut
½ tsp cinnamon
 walnuts, to decorate

This is the recipe that showed me raw food can taste as good, if not better, than the original. I haven't had normal carrot cake since trying it. Non-wheat, non-dairy and no bad refined sugar. This cake can be served as a great dessert as well. Best when kept really cold.

Lightly grease a 20cm round cake tin and line it with lightly greased baking paper.

Put all the icing ingredients in a food processor or blender and blitz until smooth. You can add a little water if the mixture appears too thick. It should be soft enough to spread.

Put all the cake ingredients in a food processor and whizz until you have a grainy, sticky mass.

Spoon half the cake mixture into the cake tin, spread it to cover the entire base of the tin and press it down firmly with the back of a spoon. Spread a third of the icing over the cake base. Put the cake tin in the freezer for about 30 minutes, until the icing has solidified.

Now pour the remaining cake mixture on top and press it down again using the back of a spoon. Then spread the remaining icing evenly over the top, again using the back of a spoon. Put the cake back in the freezer until the icing has set.

Decorate with walnuts.

INSANELY GOOD
CHOCOLATE CAKE

Makes 1 cake

For the base
150g cashew nuts
80g desiccated coconut
   or oats
60g dates
1 tbsp coconut oil, melted
salt, to taste (about ¼ tsp)

For the chocolate
   topping
3 tbsp raw cacao powder
150g cashew nuts
75ml maple syrup
2½ tbsp coconut oil,
   melted
60ml lemon juice
1 tsp vanilla essence
1 tbsp water
a little stevia, to taste, if
   you want things sweeter

As I said, I am a chocolate addict! I need to have a little bit of something chocolatey after almost every meal. This recipe is fantastic, either as a full dessert or just as a thin slice to give you that choc hit you crave!

Lightly grease a 20cm round cake tin and line it with lightly greased baking paper.

Start with the base. Put all the ingredients in a food processor and blitz until you have a sticky ball. Put into the cake tin and press down with the back of a spoon.

For the topping, blend all the ingredients until smooth. Spread the topping over the base. If you like a chunkier version, vary the blending time so there are still some crunchy nut pieces left in the mix.

Freeze for an hour before eating. After that (if anything is left), keep it in the fridge.

STRAWBERRY OR RASPBERRY CHEESECAKE

I am cheesecake-mad and the thought of giving it up would be unbearable! Luckily, thanks to this recipe, I don't have to! So, if you don't fancy the chocolate cake above, use the same recipe but leave out the chocolate and top the cake with fresh strawberries or raspberries. Amazing!

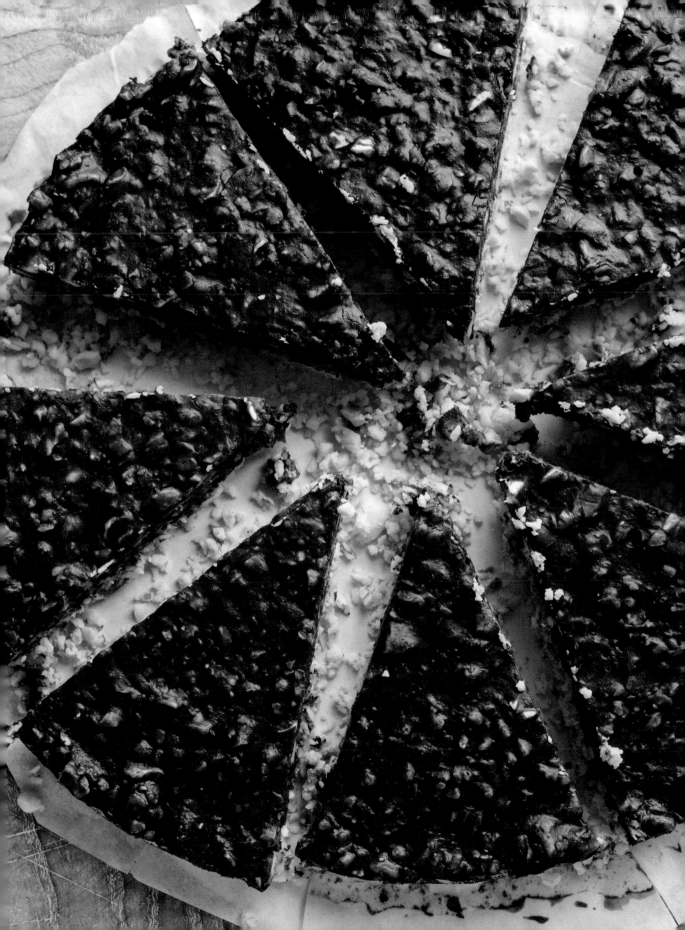

BEAR'S CHOCOLATE

For a 10 x 10cm square
1 tbsp coconut oil
1 tbsp maple syrup
2 tbsp raw cacao powder

Who knew making chocolate could be this easy and taste so darned delicious?! Rich and smooth and so satisfying. Now I sound like an advert! But it's true – this stuff tastes seriously good.

Melt the coconut oil on a low heat in a pan. Stir in the maple syrup and cacao powder.

Pour the mixture into an ice-cube tray and let it set in the freezer for 20–30 minutes until hard.

For a variation, you could add a small handful of raisins and 5 crushed walnuts to the wet mixture. Seriously good. Or add 1 tbsp desiccated coconut and a little vanilla extract.

For a completely sugar-free version, you can make this with stevia. But getting the amount right can be tricky as different brands of stevia require different measurements and the aftertaste can be bitter if you use too much. Works well with xylitol, though! And who is going to mind experimenting when it comes to tasting home-made chocolate? My family's favourite thing!

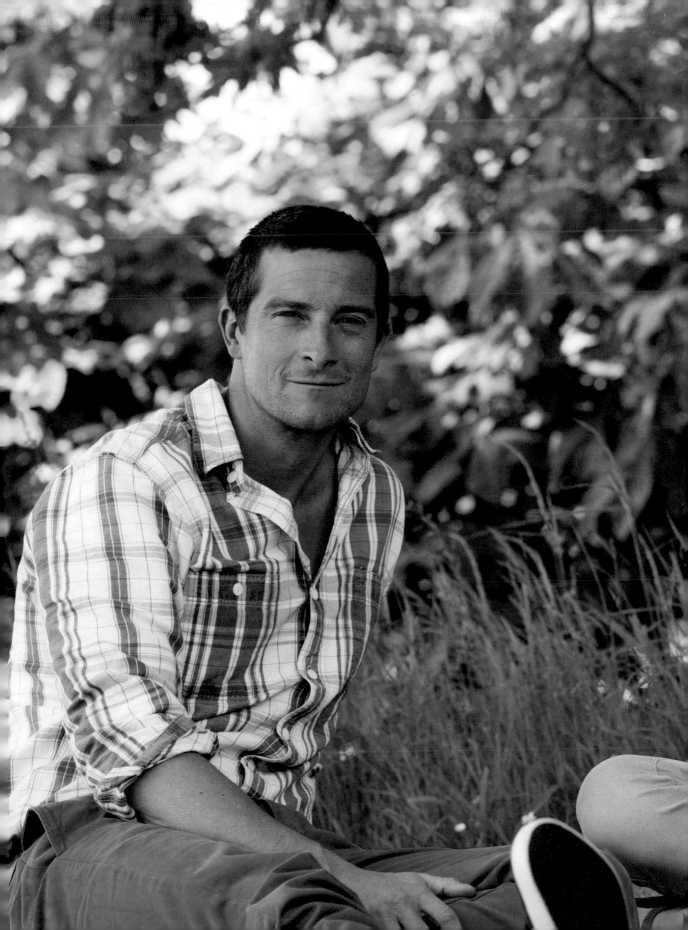

FIVE-MINUTE
CHOCOLATE BROWNIES

Makes about 10

20–30g raw cacao powder
  (more if you prefer a
  more chocolatey taste)
90g oats
150g cashews
250g dates (the stickier
  the date, the better)
2 tbsp coconut oil, melted
a pinch of sea salt

No oven needed. Made in minutes, eaten in seconds. Beware, these are highly addictive!

Put all the ingredients in a food processor, add 1 to 2 tbsp water and blitz properly until the ingredients start sticking together. You can add more water if it appears too crumbly, but only 1 tbsp at a time otherwise the mixture will go too sticky.

Put the mixture in a lightly oiled square brownie tin (about 24 x 24cm in size), spread it out and press it down gently and evenly with the back of a spoon. (If your tin is bigger or smaller, your brownies will just be thinner or thicker – don't worry about it.)

Put it in the fridge and allow to set for 30 minutes, then cut into brownie-sized pieces.

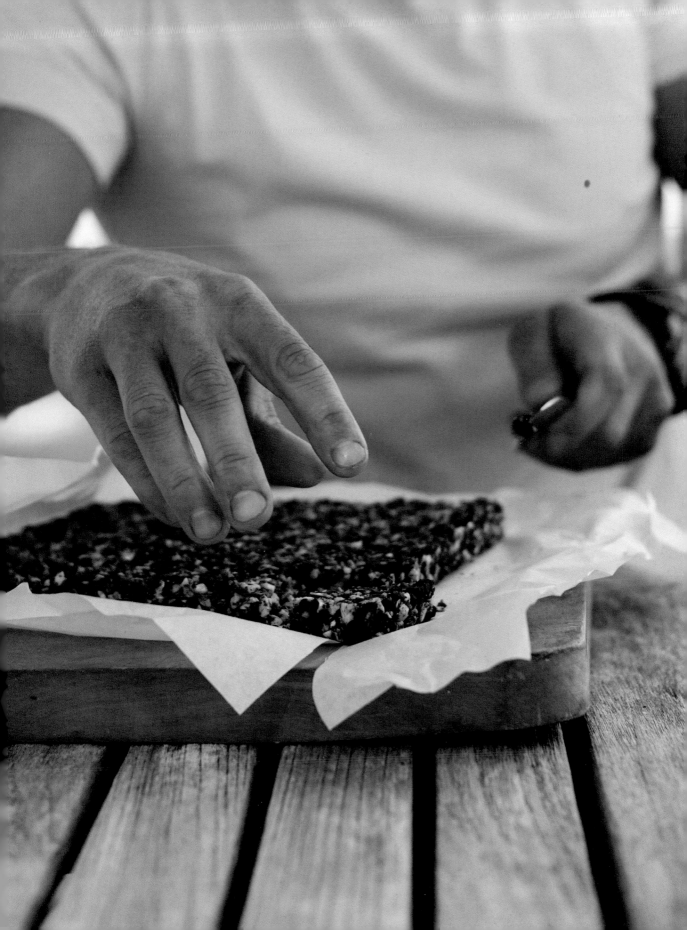

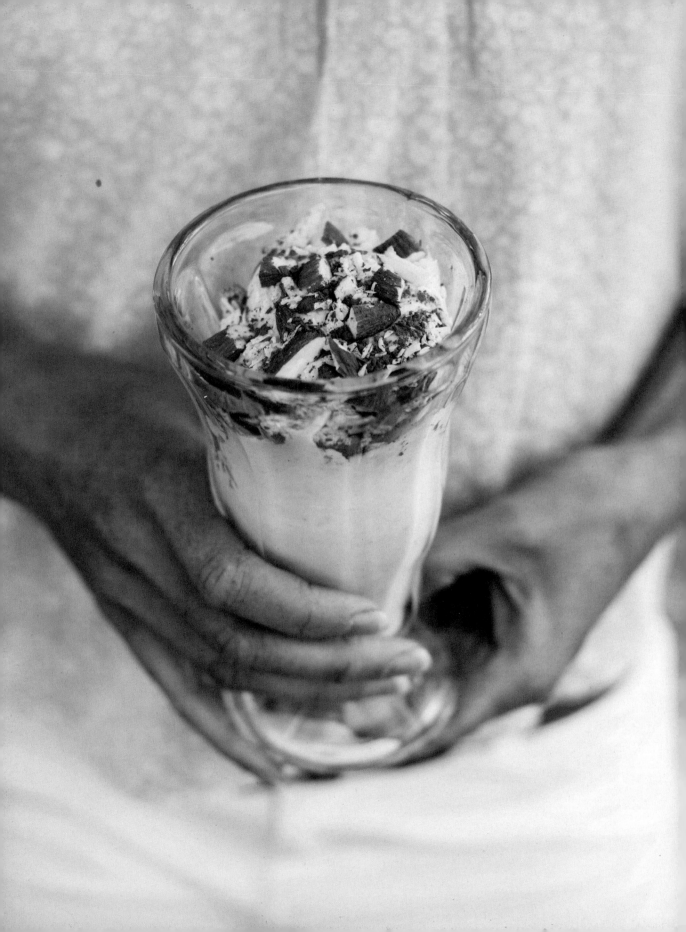

PUDDINGS

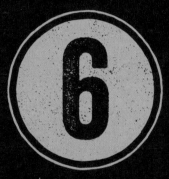

Puddings shouldn't be taken lightly! And we haven't. These recipes aren't fat- or carb-free, but we've used only wholesome, natural ingredients, including healthy oils and natural sweeteners. They are nutritional dynamite. These are still desserts, so don't go over the top, but the great thing about desserts like these is that because all the ingredients are wholesome, you feel full much faster. Anyway, enjoy, because these desserts have been both life-changing and life-enhancing for me and the family!

CHOCOLATE MOUSSE

Per person

1 egg

2 slightly heaped tbsp raw
   cacao powder

2 tbsp maple syrup

1 tbsp coconut oil, melted
   (but not hot)

a dash of vanilla essence

This chocolate mousse is incredibly good and ridiculously quick to make. If you have an unexpected guest, this is guaranteed to be a winner!

Put all the ingredients in a bowl and mix with a whisk until smooth. Spoon into a ramekin bowl.

This mousse doesn't necessarily need to set in the fridge. Just eat (with a very tiny spoon to make it last longer)!

STICKY TOFFEE PUDDING

Serves 6

For the pudding
250g dates, pitted
  and chopped
100ml rice, oat
  or almond milk
90g dairy-free butter
4 small or 3 large
  organic eggs
180g ground almonds
maple syrup, to taste
1 tsp bicarbonate of soda
1 tsp vanilla extract
a pinch of salt

For the toffee sauce
1 large tbsp dairy-free
  butter
2 tbsp palm sugar
maple syrup, to taste
230ml oat cream or
  organic soya cream
½ tsp vanilla extract
a pinch of salt

Always a firm favourite! I like mine really moist, so I don't bake it for too long, but if you like yours more sponge-like, just leave it for a little while longer. Again, guests can never believe how good this is – or that it is dairy-, wheat- and bad-sugar-free! If you grind your own almonds, leave some of them slightly roughly chopped for extra texture.

Preheat the oven to 180°C/350°F/gas mark 4. Grease 6 small pudding moulds well, or use one big dish if you prefer.

Soak the dates in 200ml boiling water for 5–10 minutes, then blend in a food processor with the remaining cake ingredients – remember that the maple syrup is the main sweetener, so adjust the quantity carefully to taste. Pour into the prepared moulds and bake to your desired firmness (anywhere between 10 and 20 minutes).

While the puddings are in the oven, make the sauce by cooking the butter, palm sugar and maple syrup on a high heat, gradually adding the cream, vanilla extract and salt to thicken.

Once the puddings are cooked, use a fork to prick them all over and pour a quarter of the sauce over them. Serve accompanied by the remaining sauce.

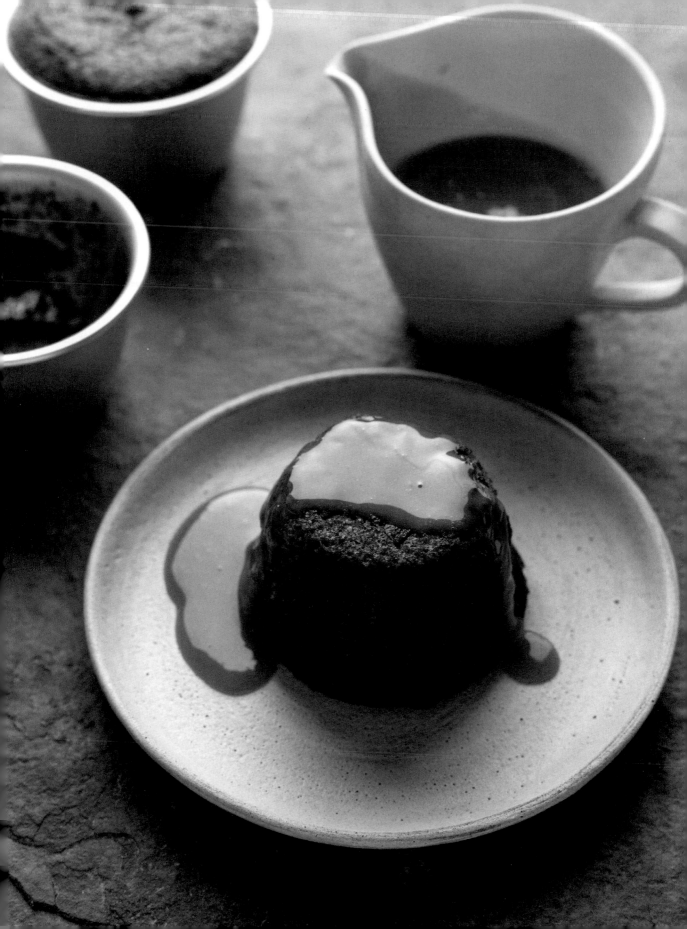

SUPER-SIMPLE
BANANA ICE CREAM

Per person
1 ripe banana
50ml coconut cream

For the topping
nuts
raw cacao powder
desiccated coconut
maple syrup

Everyone loves ice cream. Well, every kid at least. My wife, Shara, found this simple recipe while looking for what to do with some leftover bananas. Best thing about it, you don't need an ice-cream maker! Easy to make, rich and delicious, but unlike 99 per cent of ice creams, this one is super-healthy!

Take 1 ripe banana per person. Cut it into slices and freeze in an airtight container until it's completely solid to the touch (at least 2 hours).

Now transfer the banana to a food processor and add 50ml coconut cream – then start blending. First it will stay crumbly, but just keep on blending, scraping down the banana from the sides every now and again. All of a sudden, your mixture will turn white and super-creamy, just like ice cream. You can add some nuts, raw cacao powder or desiccated coconut, or drizzle a little maple syrup on the top. Endless varieties, but all healthy and 100 per cent natural.

APPLE CRUMBLE

Serves 4

80g oats

80g almond flour

100g buckwheat flour

3 heaped tbsp solid coconut
    oil (don't melt it)

2 tbsp maple syrup

salt, to taste (at least ¼ tsp)

5–6 organic apples (you can
    replace half the apples
    with berries or pears,
    if you like)

1 tsp cinnamon

a little extra coconut oil
    for greasing

After our family discovered how great buckwheat flour tasted in pancakes, we were looking for more ways of using it. Everyone loves apple crumble, right? But this one's high in fibre and protein and is all-round super-healthy. Result!

Preheat the oven to 180°C/350°F/gas mark 4. Use coconut oil to grease a 20cm ovenproof dish or 4 individual ramekins.

Mix the oats and both flours together with the coconut oil. Rub it with your fingertips into a dry crumble. Now add the maple syrup and salt. Mix and rub again until you have somewhat larger, less dry crumbles. Taste the mixture to see if you have used enough salt. It should taste great even uncooked, and definitely not bland.

Cut your apples into small pieces. Put them in a bowl and sprinkle with the cinnamon, then transfer to the prepared dish or ramekins.

Spread the crumble mixture evenly on top of the apples (if using individual ramekins, you may have a little left over) and bake for 25–30 minutes, until golden brown.

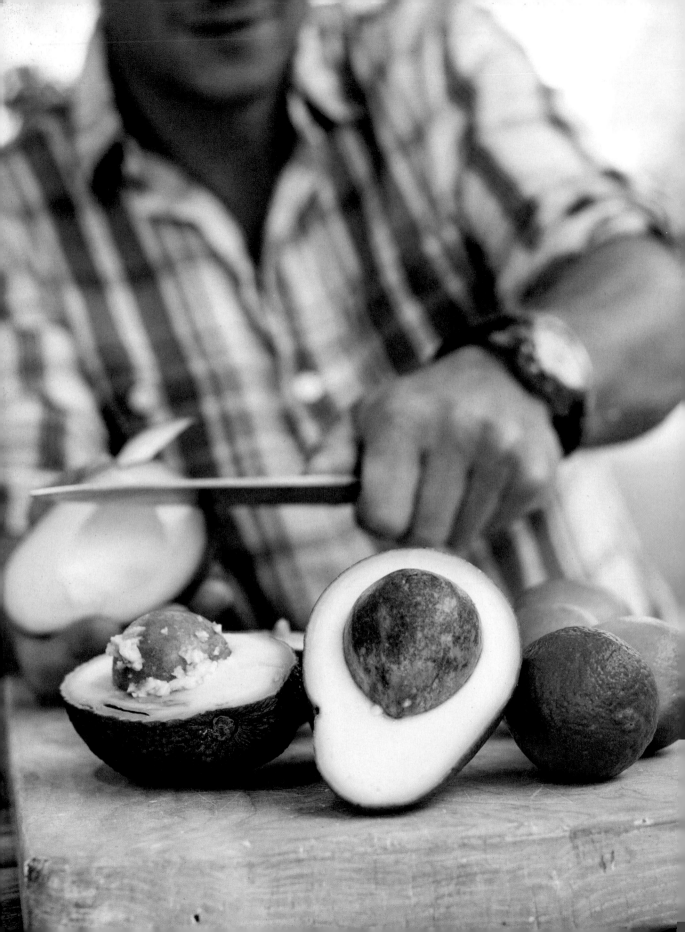

DIPS & SIDES

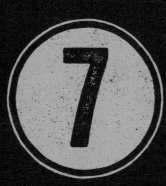

I guarantee everyone will love these, even if they're not following my nutrition plan! There are some real dinner-party winners among them.

FLAX EGGS

Flax seeds are awesome. Full of fibre. Full of omega-3 oils. Full of health-promoting nutrients. And the best thing is, you can use ground flax seeds to replace eggs in many recipes. You should buy your flax seeds whole and grind them yourself, using a coffee grinder, nut grinder or food processor. This doesn't take long but guarantees freshness and optimal health benefits. (The oils inside flax seeds are very prone to rancidity, which will make it taste very bitter and make it unhealthy.) Buy flax in bulk online, which is much cheaper and it keeps for ages. Grind enough for one week at a time and store it in the fridge in an airtight container.

To make one egg replacement, mix 1 tbsp of ground flax seeds (or you can use whole chia seeds instead) with 3 tbsp water. Let it sit for 15 minutes minimum (but no need to use immediately; it will keep for a day or two). The flax will soak up the water and become all gooey. Your flax egg is now ready to use in any recipe calling for an egg. Works great!

FOOLPROOF
GUACAMOLE

Makes 1 bowl

1 large ripe avocado

1 tbsp lime juice

1 garlic clove, skinned and finely chopped

½ small white onion, skinned and finely chopped

½ small chilli, deseeded and finely chopped

salt, to taste

An awesome dip, or great with sweet potato chips (see page 216). I mean, you haven't lived until you have had guacamole made the healthy and exotic BG way!

Cube the avocado and put a quarter of it to one side. Put the rest in a bowl with the other ingredients and mash with a fork until you have a smoothish mixture.

Now add the remaining avocado and mash again – but only a little bit, so that you still have some nice big chunks in there. Add salt to taste. Get it down you!

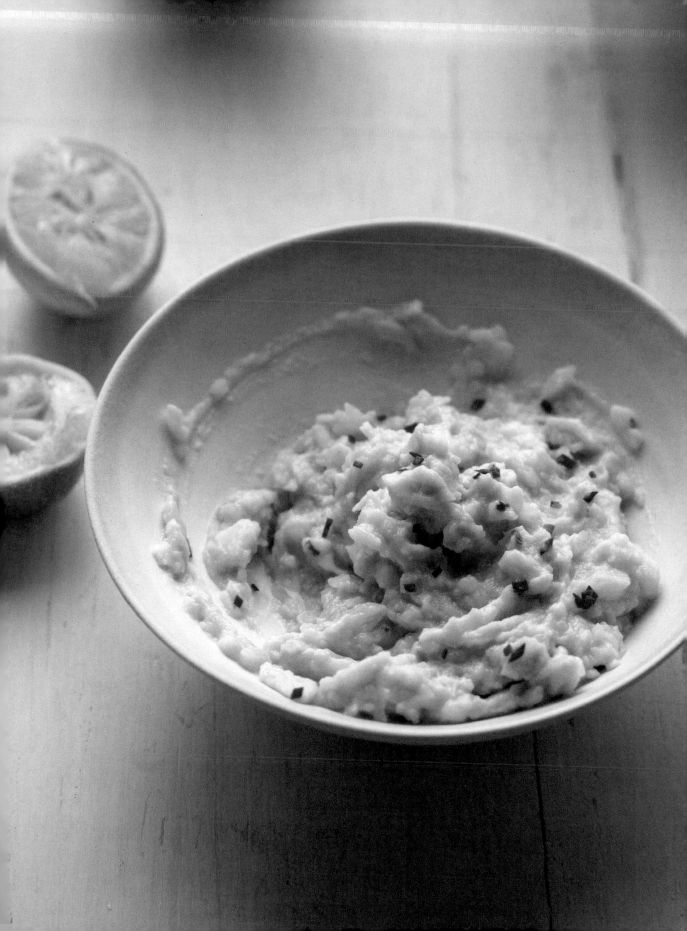

BUTTERNUT SQUASH DIP

Makes 1 bowl

½ butternut squash or a
small pumpkin (around
350g once peeled)
4 tbsp tahini
1 large garlic clove, skinned
1 tsp cumin powder
1 tsp cinnamon
juice of ½ lemon
½ tsp sea salt
pepper, to taste

**An excitingly flavoured dip which tastes fantastic
with the Super-seedy Crackers on page 210.**

Preheat the oven to 200°C/400°F/gas mark 6.

Cut the squash or pumpkin into chunks, then roast
for 30–40 minutes until soft.

Allow to cool a little then remove the peel and transfer
to a food processor (or use a hand blender) with all the
remaining ingredients and 8 tbsp water. Mix until smooth.

CAULIFLOWER POWER

Makes 1 bowl

1 head cauliflower
tinned coconut milk
1–2 garlic cloves, skinned
and crushed
salt and pepper, to taste
1–2 tbsp freshly chopped
herbs – fresh thyme and
rosemary work well

**Who needs mashed potatoes when you can make
this far healthier version? Full of fibre and flavour,
it's filling, healthy and satisfying. Great as a side
to any meat dish.**

Cut the cauliflower into florets and put them in a pan. Add
just enough coconut milk to come 2.5cm up the sides of the
pan (the cauliflower does not need to be entirely covered).

Add the garlic, salt and pepper and bring to the boil.
Simmer with a lid on until very tender, then mash with a
potato masher or in a blender. Mix in the herbs and serve
at once while still warm.

HEALTHY
HERBY BREAD

Makes 1 loaf

180g almond flour
35g ground flax seeds
   (see page 71)
1 tsp baking soda
1 tsp (not heaped)
   Himalayan crystal salt
5 eggs
1 tbsp maple syrup
1½ tbsp coconut oil, melted
1 tbsp apple cider vinegar
2 tbsp freshly chopped
   thyme leaves
2 tbsp freshly chopped
   rosemary

I have always loved bread. So to discover I could still have it but could now make it delicious and healthy was life-changing! This amazing gluten-free loaf is easy to make, delicious and filling. It comes out a little like a cake – the texture and flavour are awesome. A really good way to satisfy those bread cravings!

Preheat the oven to 175°C/350°F/gas mark 4. You'll need a bread tin about 22 x 12 x 6cm (don't worry if it's a bit larger – the loaf will just be lower). Grease it with a little coconut or olive oil.

Put the almond flour, flax seeds, baking soda and salt in a bowl and mix with a hand mixer or whisk until thoroughly combined.

Add all the remaining ingredients apart from the herbs and mix again until you have a smooth but very thick batter. Add the herbs and mix them through thoroughly.

Pour the mixture into the loaf tin – it should come about halfway up the sides. Bake for 25–30 minutes or until a toothpick inserted in the centre comes out clean and dry. Allow the loaf to cool a little, then turn it out of the tin on to a wire rack.

You can make so many different varieties of this bread. Try it with black olives and sun-dried tomatoes, or with walnuts and raisins (use only ½ tsp of salt for this). If you are allergic to eggs, use flax eggs instead (see page 201).

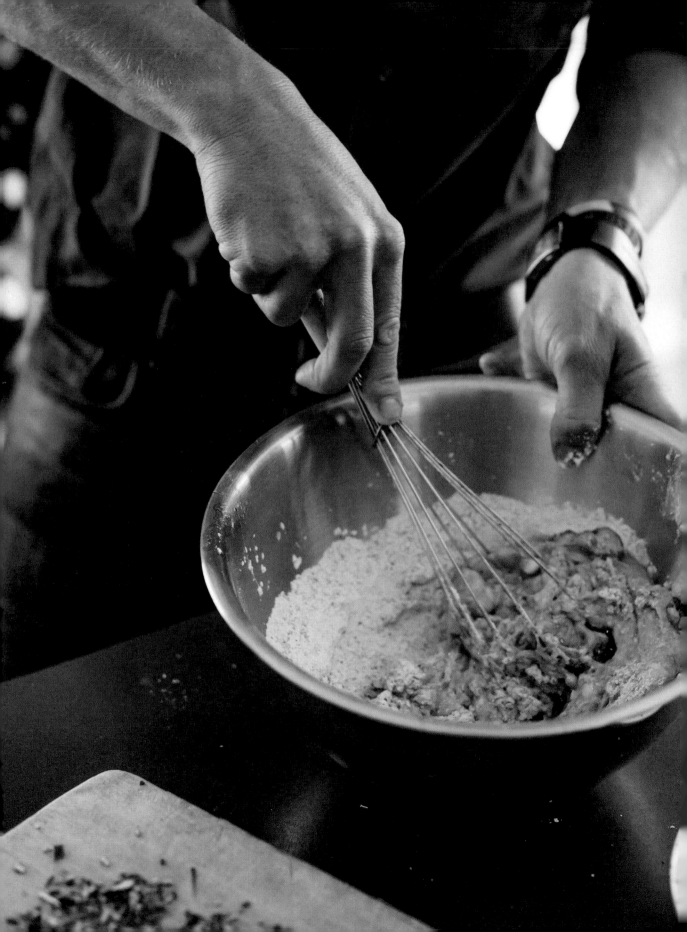

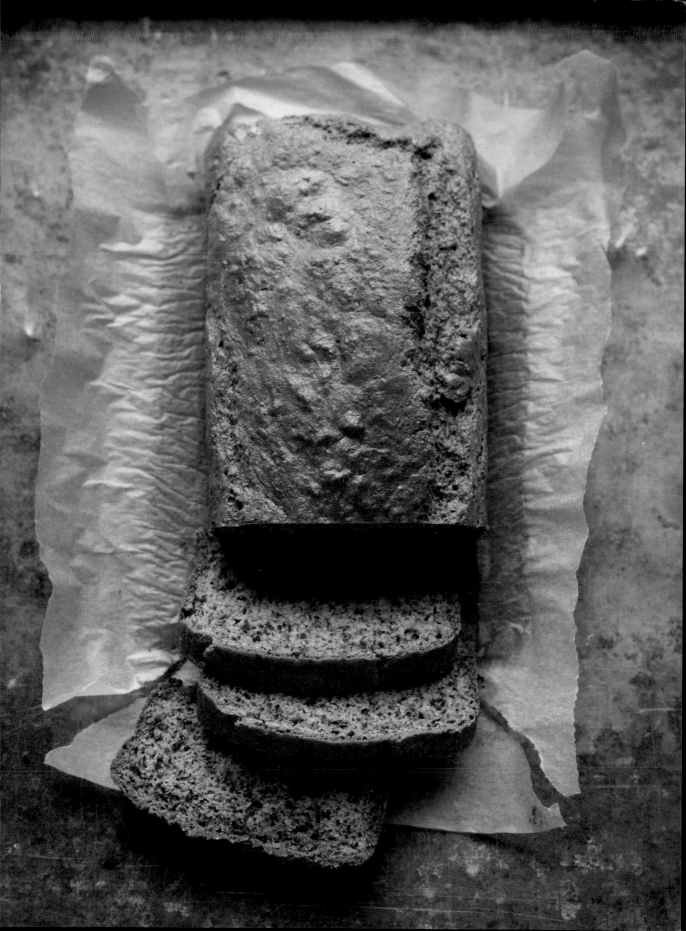

PORTOBELLO BUNS

Per bun
1 Portobello mushroom
1–2 tsp olive oil
salt and pepper

Nothing will ever properly replace a soft white burger bun – but these bread-free buns come darned close, and they are much healthier. They taste meaty, they're super-lean and they're health-enhancing. If you can grill them on a barbecue – or over a campfire – for about 5 minutes on each side instead of baking them in the oven, they taste even better!

Preheat the oven to 175°C/350°F/gas mark 4.

Don't wash mushrooms, just wipe them clean with some kitchen towel. Pour some oil on the palm of your hand and coat the outside of each mushroom.

Crack some black pepper in the middle of each mushroom along with another small drizzle of oil. (You can also add other flavours, such as some fresh chopped garlic or a sprinkle of garlic powder, chilli flakes, a dash of soy sauce, balsamic vinegar, lemon or a dash of cayenne pepper.)

Put your mushrooms on a lightly oiled baking sheet and bake for about 5–7 minutes. Alternatively, grill them for several minutes on each side. If you're grilling, start with the round side up and only add the flavours, oil and pepper when you turn them over!

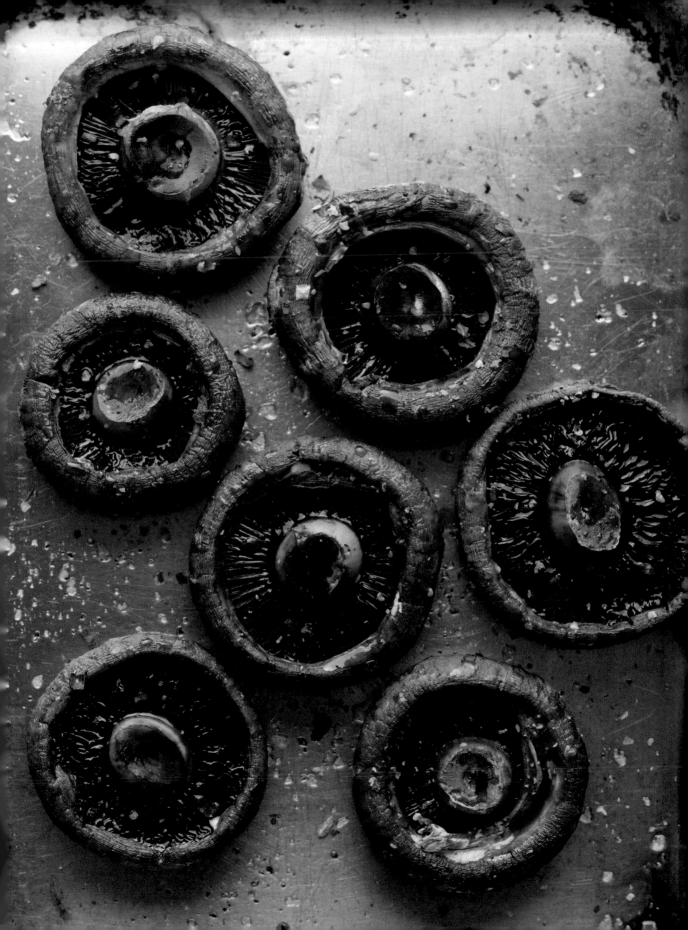

SUPER-SEEDY
CRACKERS

Makes about 12

2 parsnips, peeled
   and chopped
2 tbsp olive oil, plus
   a little extra
70g ground flax seed
   (see page 71)
½ tsp smoked paprika
   powder
½ tsp garlic powder
½ tsp cumin powder
½ tsp freshly ground
   black pepper
½ tsp Celtic sea salt
160g mixed seeds
1 tsp lemon juice

Think you don't like parsnips? Think again. These crackers are inspired! Gluten-free, egg-free, nut-free, dairy-free – great as a snack on their own, or for dipping (try them with the Butternut Squash Dip on page 204). They taste best when perfectly crisp, so oven time is essential and may need some adjusting, depending on your type of oven.

Preheat the oven to 170°C/325°F/gas mark 3½. Line a 34 x 20cm baking tray with baking paper and lightly grease it with a little olive oil.

Put the chopped-up parsnips into a food processor, together with the 2 tbsp olive oil and 6 tbsp water. Pulse until you have a very fine mixture. Add the ground flax seeds, all the spices and the salt, then pulse until properly mixed.

Transfer to a bowl and add the mixed seeds and the lemon juice and mix with your hands until you have a thick mixture.

Spread out the mixture on the baking tray and press it down using the back of a spoon. Make sure to spread the mixture evenly and as thinly as possible. With a knife, mark it into about 12 cracker-sized pieces.

Bake for 15–20 minutes. The crackers should start to brown just a little around the sides and should be entirely dry to the touch.

Remove from the oven. Put another piece of lightly oiled baking paper over the top and flip the crackers over. Now slowly peel off the old baking paper. A tiny bit of the mixture may come off – don't worry about it!

Return the crackers to the oven for another 15–20 minutes until crisp. Leave to cool for 10 minutes before removing from the baking paper.

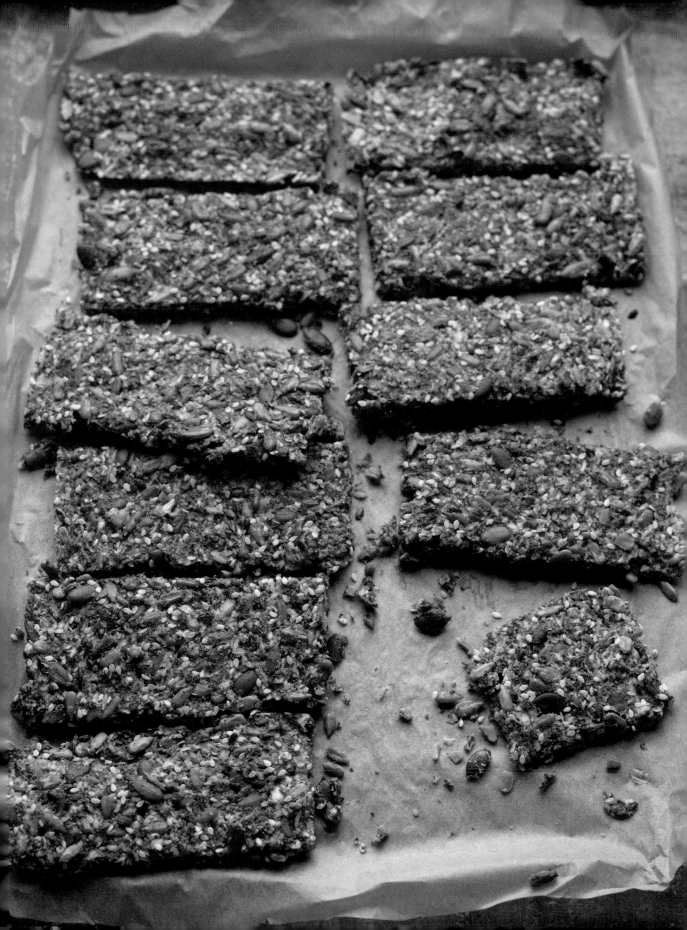

ROCKET CASHEW PESTO

Makes 1 bowl

200g unsalted cashews
2–3 tbsp (about 10g)
 nutritional yeast
1 garlic clove, skinned
100g rocket
6 tbsp olive oil
 (more to taste)
2 tbsp lemon juice
salt and pepper

Miss that bit of cheese or some cheese spread? This is a really satisfying dairy-free alternative. I love this one. It makes a brilliant dip for chunky raw veggies such as cauliflower, carrots and peppers. Works great as a pesto too!

Put the cashews, nutritional yeast and garlic in a food processor. Blitz until the ingredients are mixed but the cashews are still slightly chunky. Transfer to a bowl.

Put the rocket, olive oil and lemon juice into the food processor. Process until you have a chunky sauce.

Stir the rocket mixture into the cashew mixture, then season with salt and pepper.

If you want a more spreadable mixture, process the cashews for slightly longer and add a bit more oil. For a stronger flavour, add some extra garlic or garlic powder, or add some chilli flakes for a spicy kick.

This keeps in the fridge for up to 3 days.

DAD'S TOMATO SAUCE

Serves 2
4 organic tomatoes
a large drizzle of
    extra-virgin olive oil
a couple of garlic cloves,
    skinned
salt and lots of freshly
    ground pepper
coriander (optional)

When I was growing up, my late dad used to make this simple sauce every Sunday evening. I think it was about the only thing he could actually make, but now I understand nutrition better I see it was an inspired dish, and healthy in every respect. He always said it was a tribute to our Spanish ancestry, with its mix of olive oil, raw garlic, tomatoes and black pepper. It always tastes delicious and brings simple dishes to life. I now eat it for breakfast or as a light evening meal, served on top of either kippers or poached salmon, and with some scrambled eggs on the side. Or you could simply have it on healthy, non-wheat toast, with olive oil.

Put all the ingredients in a blender and blitz until you have a thickish sauce. You can now heat the sauce, or keep it cold.

Pour over your fish or toast.

BEAR-STYLE FRIED SWEET POTATOES

Serves 2

½ tbsp coconut oil

1 sweet potato (about 300g once peeled and cut into small cubes)

2–3 shallots, skinned and finely chopped

1 garlic clove, skinned and finely chopped

10 cherry tomatoes

½ tbsp Marmite

No more toast with Marmite for me, so I use it on my sweet potatoes instead! Tastes rich and fantastic.

Melt the coconut oil in a non-stick frying pan on medium heat and add the cubed potatoes. Fry for 5 minutes until beginning to soften.

Add the shallots, garlic, tomatoes and Marmite and stir well. Cover the pan and fry for another 5–7 minutes, stirring occasionally, until the potatoes are completely soft.

Eat straight away (but be careful – the tomatoes are red hot inside!).

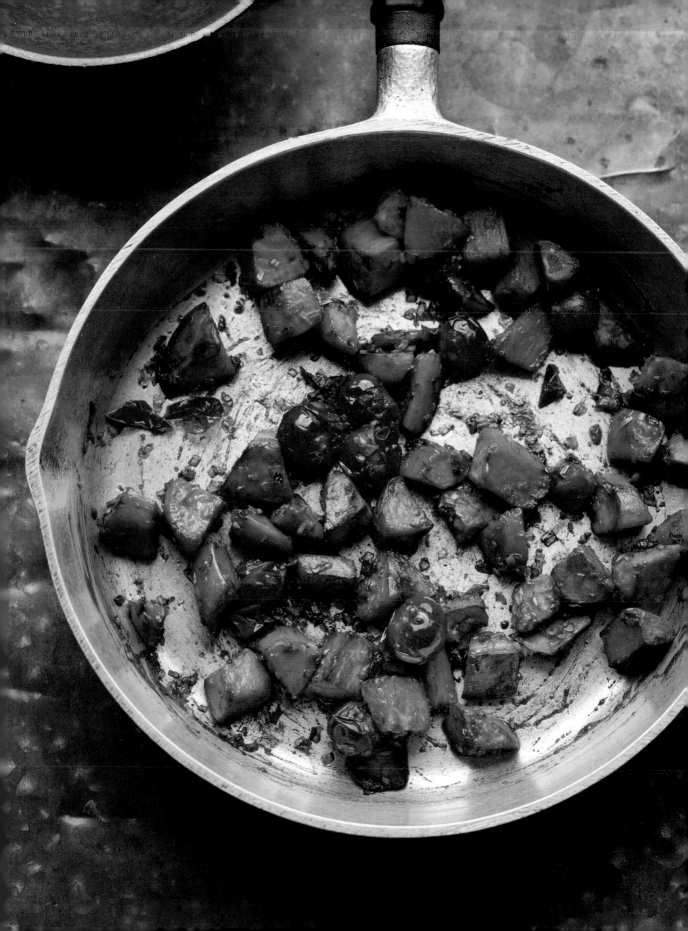

SWEET POTATO CHIPS

Per person

1 medium-sized sweet
  potato, peeled
1–2 tbsp olive oil
sea salt (about ¼ tsp)
pepper and spices of your
  choice (e.g. cayenne
  pepper, paprika, curry
  powder, garlic powder
  or cumin)
cornflour (optional)

**I've mostly ditched chips, but I do occasionally
throw in some sweet potato wedges just to scratch
that itch!**

Preheat the oven to 220°C/425°F/gas mark 7. Line a baking
tray with a non-stick baking sheet.

Cut the sweet potato into even, not too thick, chip-sized
pieces. In a bowl, mix the chips with the olive oil, salt,
pepper and spices of choice (about ½ tsp spice per potato).
To make the chips come out really crispy, sprinkle in 1 tsp
cornflour as well.

Spread the chips evenly on the baking tray and bake for 15
minutes in the upper third of your oven. Flip the chips over
with a metal spatula. Now bake for another 10–15 minutes,
until the chips are crispy, slightly browned around the
edges but still nice and soft inside.

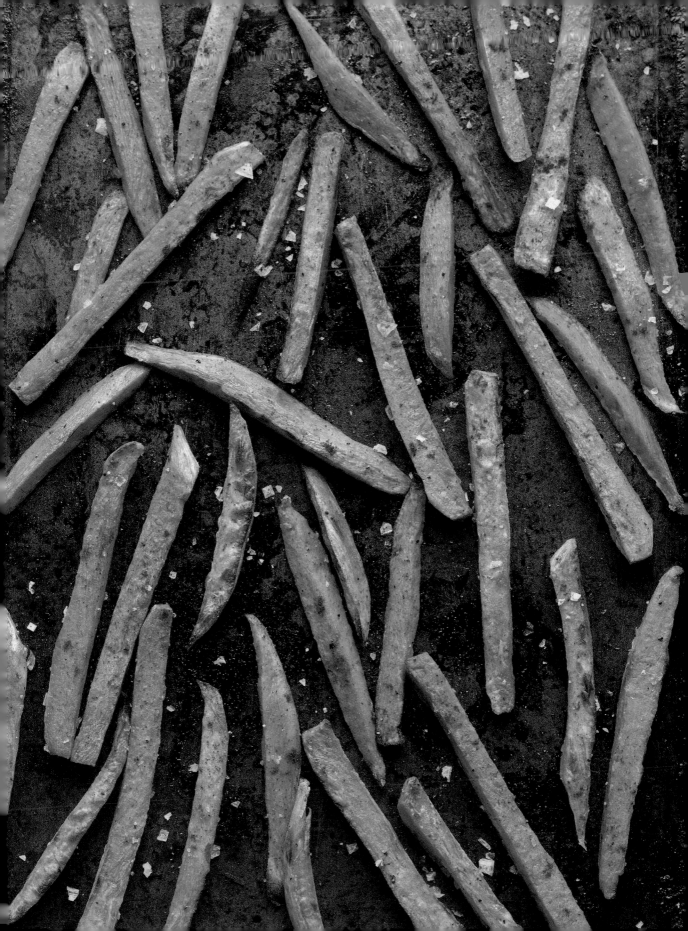

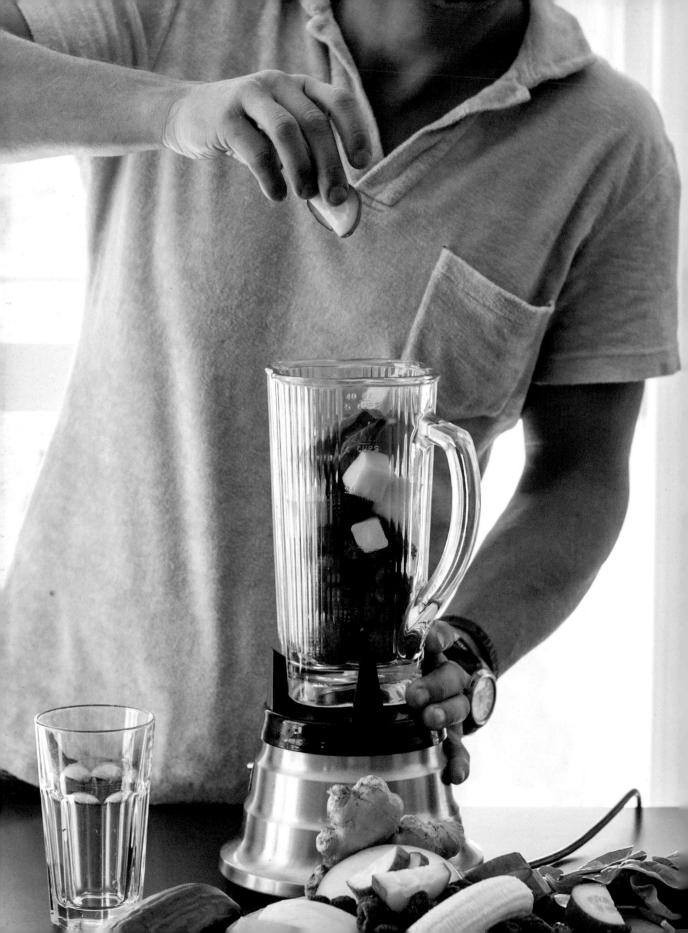

SHAKES, JUICES & SMOOTHIES

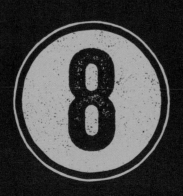

Sometimes the healthiest and simplest solution to getting a load of nutrients down you is to make a great-tasting shake, smoothie or juice. The varieties are endless, but these are some of my favourites.

I always start the day with my favourite 'clean' veggie one, in addition to the rest of my breakfast, and I will sometimes end the day with a shake as well, if I am having a 'lean' or 'fasting' day.

And I always try to have one post-workout to help restore my muscles.

SMOOTHIES

Smoothies are a versatile, tasty, nutritious and incredibly easy way to start or finish the day. They can replace a full meal if, like me, you're always in a hurry. And they make sure you touch all the nutritional bases at the start of the day when you have them for breakfast. You can make a different smoothie each day, using any of the ingredients from the list that follows.

Making smoothies is the first step to regaining control over your diet and health, and showing care for your body and mind. Start it now.

To prevent smoothies from being too carbohydrate-laden, which could affect our blood-sugar and energy levels, they should always be balanced out with *sufficient protein*. The easiest way to incorporate protein into a smoothie is by using a small scoop of protein powder. The best protein powders for health, I believe, are hemp protein, brown rice protein or pea protein. These can be bought online or in health stores. I do also use a whey protein from time to time, or when travelling, but the debate on which is healthier or better for keeping lean and supporting muscles is ongoing. As a rule of thumb, I always try to avoid whey as one of my main staples as it is derived from dairy, which we are working hard to avoid, for the many reasons discussed earlier (see pages 56–8).

All these different sources of protein powder taste slightly different. If the taste is too overpowering, use a little less until you've got used to it.

What follows is a list of base ingredients, protein sources and a few optional extras that work well in smoothies. There are so many choices – it is a matter of your personal taste which of them you use. Simply blitz your ingredients in a blender or food processor, and make the smoothie thicker or thinner by adjusting the quantity of liquid you use. After that, a few of my favourite smoothie recipes.

Smoothies are great (and important) after exercise to replace lost nutrients, fluid and glucose, and to provide your muscles with much-needed protein.

BUILD YOUR OWN SMOOTHIE

Base ingredients

Any fruits. Berries, mango, banana and papaya work especially well. ½ cupful fruit should do (you can use more for a sweeter taste).

Any nuts or seeds, such as chia seeds, flax seeds, pumpkin seeds, almonds, walnuts, pecan nuts and Brazil nuts – vary the types. Use around 2 tbsp. Instead of nuts you can also use 1 large tbsp nut or seed butter, such as almond butter, cashew butter or sunflower seed butter.

Rather than ordinary milk, use a dairy replacement such as oat milk, almond milk, coconut milk, hemp milk, coconut yoghurt, organic soya milk or yoghurt. (I mostly use oat or almond milk.) Use as much as you need to get the consistency you want (some like their smoothies thick, some like them more liquid.)

Add a handful of organic raw spinach – it doesn't affect the taste, only the colour! Other vegetables that taste mild and work well are cooked beetroot or grated courgette.

You can add a drizzle of oil such as hemp oil or flax oil. These are especially beneficial if you do not eat fish.

A spoonful or two of oats (this makes the smoothie thicker).

A generous sprinkle of cinnamon, if you like the taste (this helps to balance blood sugar).

Use stevia, maple syrup, xylitol or raw honey to sweeten if your smoothie isn't sweet enough. (I use stevia as it is natural and calorie-free.)

Protein sources
Choose from:
½ avocado (neutral in taste but gives smoothies body)
protein powder, 1–2 tbsp per smoothie

Extras
desiccated coconut
raw cacao powder
baobab powder, maca powder, lucuma powder or wheatgrass powder (bought in health shops or online)
fresh mint leaves

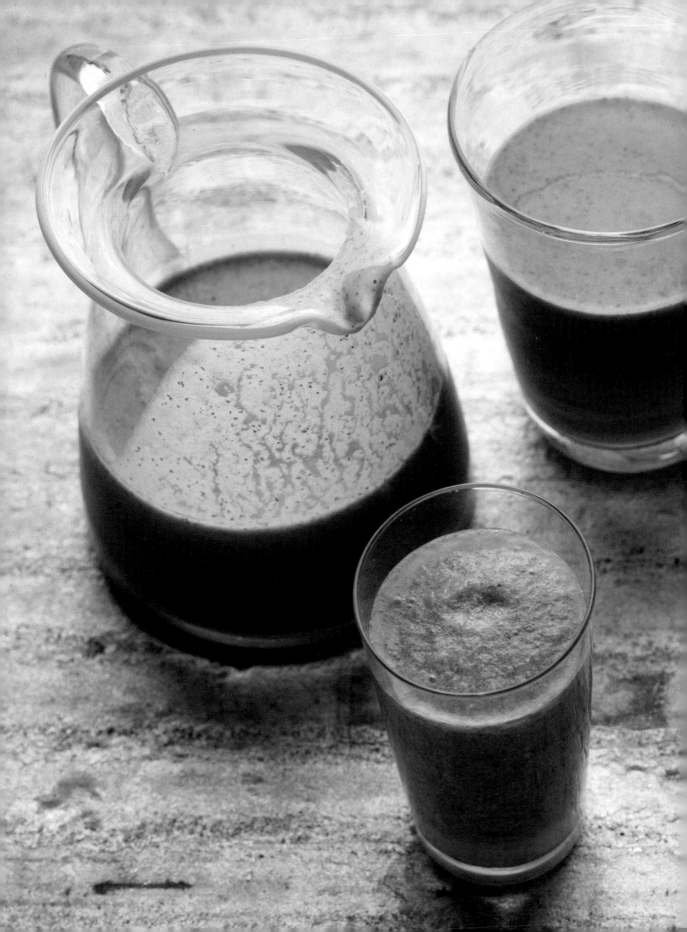

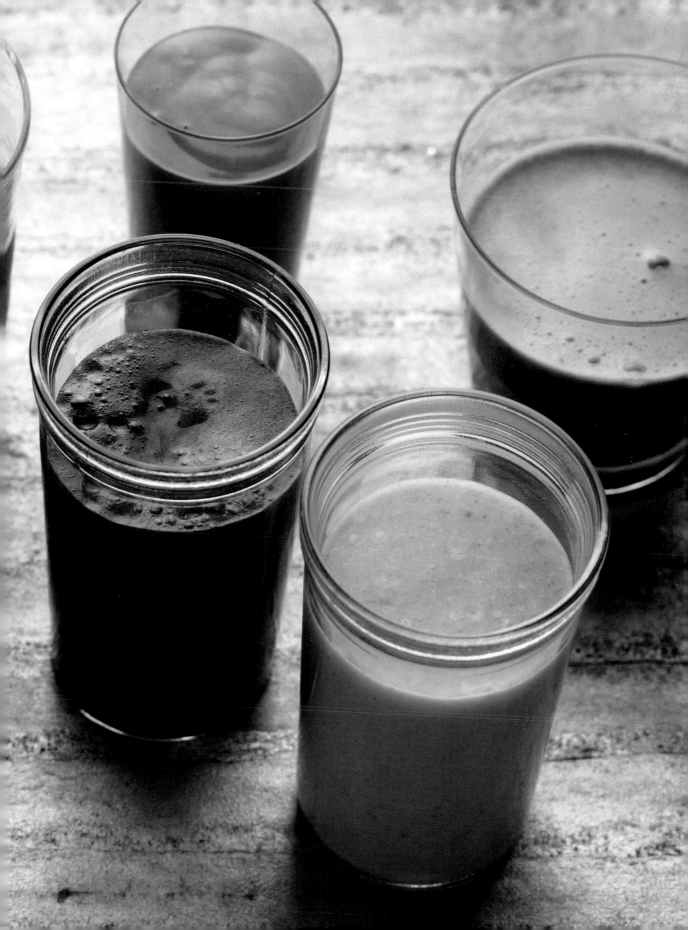

BEAR'S POST-WORKOUT SMOOTHIE 1

almond milk
1–2 tbsp protein powder
    (hemp, rice or pea)
½ banana
a small handful of berries
    (strawberries/raspberries/
    blueberries)
stevia, to sweeten
1 tbsp chia seeds
an optional handful
    of oats

BEAR'S POST-WORKOUT SMOOTHIE 2

coconut milk
1 ripe banana
1 tbsp pumpkin seeds
¼ tsp vanilla extract
1 tsp honey or maple syrup
2 tsp almond butter
1–2 tbsp protein powder
a sprinkle of cinnamon
optional: a large handful of organic baby-leaf
    spinach and a pinch of turmeric

BEAR'S POST-WORKOUT SMOOTHIE 3

oat milk, coconut milk, hemp milk or water
1 orange, peeled
6 frozen mango pieces or ½ fresh mango,
    chopped
a large handful of spinach
1 tbsp cashew butter
1–2 tbsp protein powder

HIDDEN VEG SMOOTHIE

almond milk
1 small courgette, grated
2 large handfuls of blueberries
2 large handfuls of spinach
1 tbsp flax or chia seeds
1 tbsp cashew butter
natural sweetener to taste (1–2 dates, coconut
    palm sugar, stevia or maple syrup)

BEAR'S FAVOURITE MORNING SHAKE 1

ice or water to blend
½ cucumber, skin still on
a small handful of mint
1 carrot, chopped
a couple of broccoli florets
2 cm piece of ginger (or more!)
½ lemon
½ pear, apple or orange

BEAR'S FAVOURITE MORNING SHAKE 2

almond milk
1 banana
1 tbsp chia seeds
2 tbsp oats
ice
stevia to sweeten

IMMUNE-BOOSTING SHAKE

almond milk
2cm piece fresh turmeric
   (or ½ tsp dried turmeric)
2.5cm piece of ginger, peeled
1 banana
¼ pineapple, cut into chunks
1 tsp vanilla extract

CHOCOLATE BANANA SHAKE

1 ripe banana, chopped and then frozen
1 heaped tsp cacao powder
1–2 tbsp almond butter
almond milk
natural sweetener, to taste (xylitol, coconut
   palm sugar, stevia or maple syrup)
½ tbsp chia seeds
a dash of cinnamon
a handful of crushed ice

PINT OF SALAD

3–4 broccoli florets
juice of 1 lime
a handful of parsley
1 sweet apple, peeled
    and chopped
2 handfuls of spinach
a little stevia, if it isn't
    sweet enough

A great way to get in a load of greens without having to cook. OK, so for a week, whenever you get a craving to head for the snack cupboard, make this first and see if you still fancy a snack afterwards! Try it. It's a fun and revealing experiment in how our minds and bodies actually work.

Put all the ingredients in a blender with some water (start with 200ml) and blitz until you have a shake. Make it as thick or thin as you like by adding more or less water. Drink immediately.

JUICING/BLENDING

If you have a powerful blender or a juicer, always stick to the 80:20 ratio. This means 80 per cent vegetable juice (preferably green), 20 per cent fruit juice. Remember that apples, pears, ginger, lemon and melons help make your juices taste fruity and zesty, even if you put tons of greens in. Carrots also help to sweeten it.

To be honest, I very rarely juice now – I tend always to blend. I throw everything – skin, core and all – into a powerful blender on max power, and blitz it into a delicious purée drink. This gives me all the fibre and goodness that juicing loses.

Here are two easy and tasty purée/juice examples.

GREEN JUICE

2 large handfuls of kale
½ cucumber
2 celery stalks
2 pears
½ lemon
2.5cm piece of ginger

PRE-WORKOUT JUICE

4 carrots
1 cucumber
1 beetroot
2 large handfuls of spinach
½ lemon
2 small or 1 large sweet apple

EASY SUGAR-FREE
LEMONADE

Makes 1 jug

750ml bottle naturally
    carbonated spring water
2 tsp stevia (adjust to taste,
    and according to the
    brand)
freshly squeezed lemon
    juice, to taste
chopped-up strawberries,
    to taste

Who needs sugary or artificially sweetened drinks when you can make a great, sweet, fizzy lemonade at home, bursting with flavour and vitamins! There are endless varieties, but this is how I make mine.

Just mix all the ingredients in a jug. Play around with the amounts to create your perfect sweetness, and feel free to add any other fruit you like.

Another great combo is lemon, cucumber, mint, apple and orange – a bit like Pimm's without the alcohol! (My kids love to eat up all the fruit with a spoon or straw.)

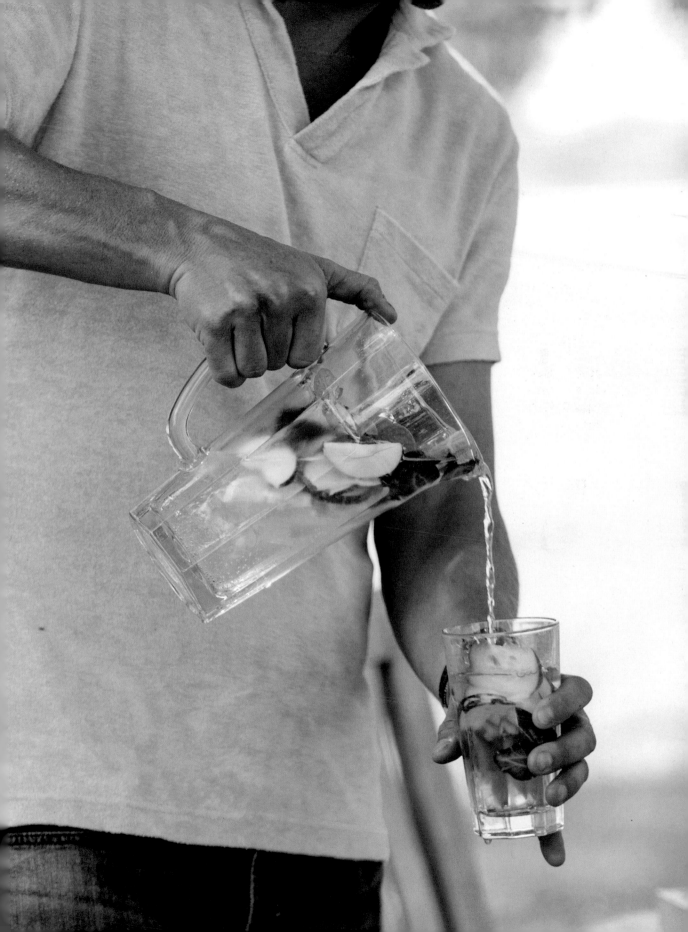

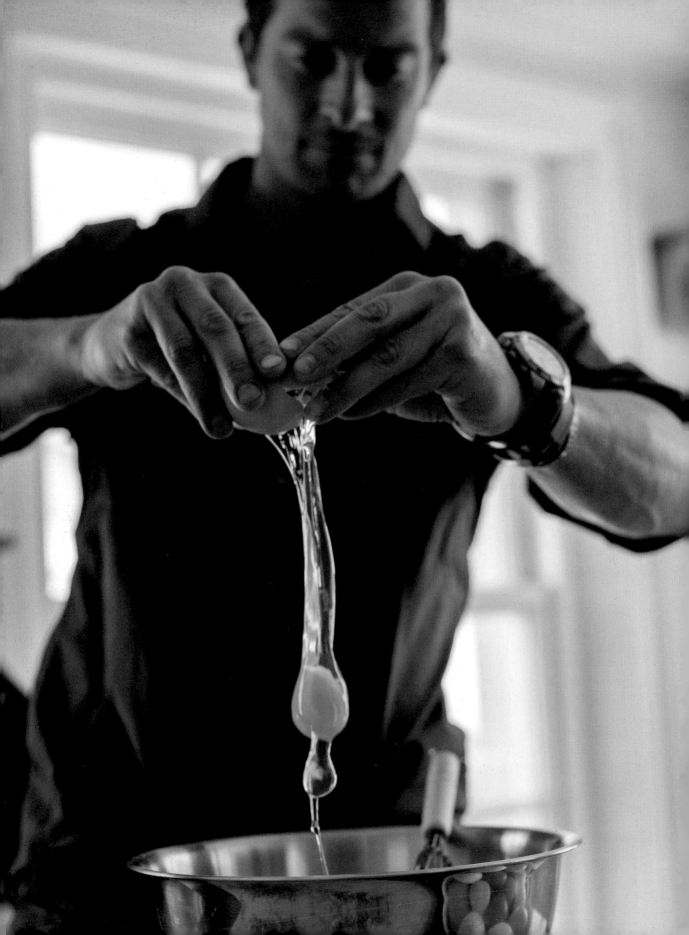

GO
FOR
IT!

8-WEEK EATING PLAN

What follows is my no-nonsense 8-week eating plan for ultimate health and maximum energy.

If you've got this far in the book, hopefully you're beginning to understand why I choose to eat the way I do. It makes me feel energized, healthy and ready for anything that the world (and the wild) throws at me.

But I know that changing the way you think about food can be daunting. It was for me too. It's not going to happen overnight, and chances are you're going to need a bit of a helping hand. That's where my eating plan comes in.

You can think of what follows as a temporary try-out plan – a way of dipping your toe into the water. Or you can think of it as a plan to change your entire lifestyle. Either way, I recommend that you keep it up for 80 per cent of the time and treat yourself for 20 per cent of the time – see page 15 for more on the 80:20 rule.

Eight weeks is a decent amount of time to make all the necessary changes for the average person. However, if you want to do it faster or slower, that is totally fine. Don't feel that the eight-week thing is a straightjacket. If you aren't a coffee drinker, or you already don't eat gluten, you'll be able to make the plan several weeks shorter. If all the changes come easily to you, you might be able to make it as short as three or four weeks. Alternatively, if you find it trickier, just take it more slowly and spread the plan over several weeks more. There are no hard rules on timing. What works for someone else might not work for you. Ease yourself in, and as you see your body changing, your health improving and your family responding to new, delicious-tasting recipes, take on a little more.

And don't beat yourself up if you fall off the wagon. Remember: failure is just a step on the path to success! Nobody ever achieved anything worthwhile without failing a whole load of times first. So, be kind to yourself. Just dust yourself down and throw yourself back into the fray. It's normal to have blips. Just remember: keep them as blips, not flatliners!

This is a marathon, not a sprint. It is the journey for the rest for your life, to build health, fitness and longevity.

It isn't an all-out race to blow out, after which you then fall back to your old ways. This book is your re-education! Embrace it and be prepared to have your eyes opened wide in terms of what is healthy and how to cook it deliciously. That's the goal.

The information in this book is incredible – truly – and I don't just say that because Kay and I wrote it! It really can be life-changing and life-enhancing. So much of life is about the enjoyment of great-tasting food. I don't want to write a book of wacky recipes that taste bland and which no one sticks with beyond ninety days of experimenting! This is about changing you for the better, leaner and healthier.

And remember: very little in this plan involves giving up anything, as we have worked so hard to find amazing alternatives! This is true of the wheat, the sugar, the salt and the dairy. So, if you do it right and follow the recipes and principles, and also keep putting into your brain the empowering knowledge of what the good stuff gives and what the bad stuff takes from you, it really should be straightforward and achievable.

This isn't Everest. I know that you are busy out there climbing your own mountain in your work or personal life already, whether you are a single parent or trying to be a CEO. Everyone is fighting their own battles. I simply want this to be achievable and empowering. I want this plan simply to be that positive re-education that will fuel you better for climbing whatever mountains you are aiming for in the rest of your life. And for the journey to be delicious along the way!

And ultimately, remember that if you are crumbling – hey, have your cheat meal! Go eat a pizza! Then get back on track.

Track your progress
I truly believe that following this 8-week plan can make you feel healthier, less stressed and more energized. But as these changes happen gradually, it can be easy to miss how dramatic they are. That's why you should keep track of your progress. I think you'll be amazed by the effects your new way of eating can have.

To do this, fill out the following short questionnaire before you start the plan. Do it again after four weeks and finally at the end of the eight weeks.

HOW IS YOUR HEALTH?

1. Your current weight ▢

2. Your mood over the past several weeks

Happy ▢
Anxious ▢
Irritable ▢
Depressed ▢
Aggressive ▢
Hyperactive ▢

3. Your overall stress levels on a scale from 1 to 10 ▢
(1 = very stressed, 10 = not at all stressed)

4. Your overall energy levels throughout the day, on a scale from 1 to 10
(1 = no energy, 10 = loads of energy)

Mornings: ▢

Afternoons: ▢

Evenings: ▢

5. Your digestion in the past week (1 = terrible, 10 = no issues) ▢

Regular bowel movements ▢
Bloating ▢
Flatulence ▢
Acid problems ▢

Other digestive issues ▢

6. Your sleep over the past week ▢
(1 = hardly slept at all, 10 = slept well all night)

7. Write down any other physical symptoms you have, for example arthritis, acne or haemorrhoids, and note down their severity
(1 = as bad as could be, 10 = as good as could be).

▢ ▢

WEEK 1: FOCUS ON FLUIDS

When people think about diet, they often focus solely on food. But if you've read the chapter on fluids – and if you've spent any amount of time in the wild – you'll know that fluids are vital to your health.

So, a nice easy start. Think of it as a gentle walk in the foothills before you tackle the main peak. We're going to kick off by making sure you're putting the right sort of liquid fuel in the tank.

To do this, we're gradually going to phase out caffeinated drinks and sugary/artificially sweetened drinks.

Possible side effects this week include headaches, slight drowsiness and irritability from caffeine/sugar withdrawal.

Caffeine

If you can just kick the caffeine – think coffee, black tea, Coke and 'energy' drinks – then great. There's a chance, however, that when you cut out caffeine quickly, you may experience headaches and low energy. These are temporary. They are signs that your body is overcoming your addiction. Push on through!

If you drink a ton of caffeine, though, you might find these withdrawal symptoms particularly tough. That's totally OK. Nobody climbs Everest or rows across the Atlantic without taking some smaller steps first. That's exactly what we're going to do.

Instead of doing this over the first week, do it over several. And the best way to do it is to keep a caffeine diary.

Tea Alternatives

We Brits love a cup of tea. I was pretty addicted to endless cups of builder's tea during the day, from years back, starting with my military days (NATO issue: hot, sweet tea drunk all through whatever we were doing every day!). So it was ingrained deep. I didn't want to change suddenly to some herbal, smelly tea – that would have been a terrible replacement! Then I found a perfect substitute: red bush tea with a splash of oat milk. It looks like normal tea – hot, brown and wet (NATO issue through and through!). It tastes delicious, and is super-healthy.

There are hundreds of other black-tea alternatives.

CAFFEINE DIARY

Week 1 Make a note of all the caffeine you drink per day for 7 days straight, then work out the average number of drinks per day. For example, if you drink 35 caffeinated drinks in a week, you're averaging 5 per day.

Week 2 Cut your daily intake by 1 cup a day (or 2 if you can). So instead of 5 drinks a day, you now have only 4 (or 3). You can replace the other drinks with herbal teas, coffee alternatives, fresh juices, shakes or water (see pages 46, 84, 219–30).

Week 3 Cut your daily intake down again by 1-2 drinks, once more replacing it with herbal teas, coffee alternatives, fresh juices, shakes or water.

Keep doing this until you are down to 1 (or preferably zero) caffeinated drink a day. You will most likely notice a change (for the positive!) in your energy levels, your waistline and your digestive health.

In the wild you can make brilliant, healthy teas from roots, barks and herbs (check out my book *Extreme Food* for more on that). At home, it's a bit easier! My favourite herbal teas are **red bush (rooibos)**, **fennel**, **peppermint**, **ginger**, **cinnamon** and **camomile**. Or you could try sliced or grated ginger with boiling water poured over – it makes a super-healthy tea with no tea bag! If you miss the taste of coffee, check out the alternatives on pages 82–3. Or try dandelion root coffee or chicory coffee, which look like coffee and are great for digestion and detoxification. Replace your lattes and cappuccinos with a cup of Nature's Horlicks (page 180).

Sugary drinks

Replace sugary drinks with the nourishing shakes and juices in the recipe section (see pages 219–30).

Another great way to replace fizzy, sugary drinks is to make home-made lemonade. It's cheap and easy – see page 230. Or make a big jug of fresh berries, slices of apple, mint and naturally carbonated water. The varieties are endless and kids will love trying to get out the berries with a straw!

You can also opt for coconut water or beetroot juice. Excellent exercise fluids.

Alcohol

I'm not teetotal and you don't have to be either. But you should reduce alcohol intake to a healthy level. If you're following the 80:20 rule, you can allow yourself a couple of cheat meals a week – but don't binge-drink on those! That is the one thing that research shows really does long-term damage. Be smart: drink in moderation. That is the best way anyway. No one likes a drunk! A few glasses of wine is great and sociable, but leave it there. That's enough to get all the pleasure without any of the downside.

Always think quality over quantity. Much better to have a glass of decent, organic wine than a whole bottle of plonk. I don't mean that the wine has to be fancy, expensive and from some weird chateau! Just use the internet to research healthy wines – it can actually be quite fun. And don't be peer-pressured into drinking more than you want. People respect strength and a strong will. Drink socially but be disciplined. Your peers will probably either envy you or want to copy you. (I call this reverse peer pressure.)

Water

Make it a ritual to have a pint of lukewarm water with a squeeze of fresh lemon juice the moment you get up in the morning. This will help flush out all the toxins that have accumulated overnight; it also helps you go to the loo and kick-starts your digestion. A simple step that has great health benefits.

If you want to do the same as me, find a great artesian-acquifer bottled-water brand that is rich in all the positive minerals and ideally has zero nitrates. This means it will be mega-pure and health-enhancing. Avoid the un-ecological brands or the bottled-water companies that are ground-water sourced – or even worse, that just sell de-chlorinated tap water! Failing that, go with filtered water – just make sure you change the filters regularly as bacteria can build up.

Follow the rule of checking the colour of your urine (see page 44) and top up with more glasses of water where necessary.

START YOUR DAY

Understand that in these first few weeks we are beginning to break some deep-rooted habits! They reckon it takes 21 days to form or break a habit. Many of your sugary drinks or caffeine addictions have been with you for years, maybe decades, so anticipate some hurdles, some conflicts, some struggles and some failures. You may lose a few battles along the way, but we are going to win the war for a healthier, leaner, fitter you! So, hang on in there – 21 days and you can form yourself some positive new habits. And after eight weeks – that's only 56 days – those positive new habits will be well entrenched! But this is just your warning order: anticipate some trials in these early days. And consider them a sign that you have begun a journey of some distinction!

WEEK 2: CUTTING OUT DAIRY

By dairy, at this stage in the plan, we're mainly talking milk, cream and yoghurt, which you can easily replace with non-dairy alternatives. Don't worry too much if you're still eating butter and cheese – we'll deal with those later.

Cutting out these dairy items might seem like a chore, but it really isn't. If you've read the chapter on dairy, you'll know that there are lots of alternatives to milk, cream and yoghurt. Try some of them out. Experiment. Be open-minded. (Remember – your mind is like a parachute: it works best when open!) There are loads of healthy non-dairy alternatives, many available at your supermarket. For example: **hemp milk**, **almond milk**, **hazelnut milk**, **coconut milk** (in a carton or in a tin), **coconut cream** (in a tin or dried in a block), **oat milk**, **oat cream**, **organic soya milk**, **organic soya cream**, **rice milk**, **soya yoghurt** and **coconut yoghurt**. Make sure to check the ingredients – some of these have added sugar or syrup. Try to pick the ones that don't.

Don't give up after the first try. These alternatives can taste quite different from actual dairy, but you'll soon get used to the flavour. Find the one you like the most. Let your kids find their favourite. You can have a different one each week!

Quite a few of the recipes in this book use coconut milk or cream. If you don't like the flavour, change it for soya cream, plain soya yoghurt or oat cream. They work just as well.

SHARE THE LOAD

When embarking on any ambitious project, especially one as personal as food, which is linked to our moods and our childhood habits, it makes such a difference to have a friend or family member with whom you can go through it. It helps you to keep motivated and inspired, gives you someone with whom to talk through ideas, share your struggles and plan the route ahead. You can also keep each other going when you feel like giving up. I would say this is one of the key lessons I have learned in the wild and in the many ambitious projects I have undertaken, with colleagues, friends or family: the understanding that together we are always stronger.

WEEK 3: CHEESE

So you've got this far? Awesome. I bet you're feeling pretty great already. Time to step things up a bit.

I'm not going to lie: Week 3 is a tough one, especially for hardcore cheese eaters like I was! But cheese is dairy and therefore we choose not to have it, for so many reasons. Just avoiding the huge number of unnecessary calories that are packed into even a small amount of cheese will be enough to make you way trimmer. So look at this as a positive step to getting fitter. If you have read my chapter on dairy (pages 56–8), you'll totally get why it's not a great thing, so re-read that whenever you need reminding.

If you find this hard to do and want an in-between solution, goat's cheese can be OK for the occasional non-cheat meal. Most people generally find goat's milk easier to digest than cow's milk.

However, if you are going to follow this plan fully and cut out all types of cheese – as I recommend for maximum glowing health and longevity – it is good to have some tasty alternatives to put on your bread. (In Weeks 5 and 6 you're going to cut out gluten, but these are just as good on gluten-free breads or crackers.) Here are some options:

- **Hummus** – versatile, comes in many different flavours and mixes well with salads of all kinds. Not just great as a dip, but also spread on healthy bread with some added green leaves.

- **Rocket Cashew Pesto** – see page 212.

- **Avocado** – spread ripe avocado on to your bread with a pinch of Himalayan salt and some freshly cracked pepper, or try the Foolproof Guacamole recipe on page 202.

- **Nut or seed butters** – don't be put off by the word 'butter': these spreads don't contain any dairy. There are so many varieties these days, such as pumpkin-seed butter, almond butter and cashew butter. They are a far healthier option than cheese. Most supermarkets sell a decent variety, health shops sell even more.

● **Cheese-free pestos** (to make your own, use any pesto recipe and replace the cheese with nutritional yeast flakes).

I've already mentioned **nutritional yeast** in the Milk and Dairy chapter (see page 56). I found it helped a lot, and I'm a bit of a convert. If, like me, you really miss that cheesy flavour in sauces, pestos and the like, give it a go. Although most of the recipes in this book can be made by shopping at your local supermarket, please make an extra trip to a health shop, or buy several jars of nutritional yeast online. It's sold in flake or powder form, is cheap, and not only does it help to create that cheesy taste, it really packs a punch of nutrients too (B vitamins and protein, for example). Don't worry if you can't tolerate yeast: this type won't affect you and is fine to eat.

To see how great this stuff is, try the Mediterranean Quiche on page 142, or the Cashew Lasagne on page 156, which taste amazing even without cheese. Or try making a cheese-free parmesan by mixing ¼ cup nutritional yeast with ⅓ cup raw almonds and a pinch of salt in a food processor.

Of course, these alternatives will never taste *exactly* like cheese, but they are a satisfying, healthy alternative in dairy-free dishes.

COMMITMENT IS KEY

Changing the way you eat is always going to be a challenge. But worthwhile things never come easy. If it was easy, obesity, diabetes and bloatedness wouldn't be so prevalent. Eating badly is so easy. Learning to fuel yourself and sticking to it takes time, dedication and commitment. But the prize at the end is really worth it. Eight weeks in and you will be so in the groove of healthy living, you will feel better, be fitter, trimmer and will be enjoying amazing recipes that leave you feeling full. You won't want to go back to your old ways! But to get there will take some commitment and some perseverance. My mum used to say: 'Commitment is doing the thing you said you would do long after the mood you said it in has left you!' Smart lady.

WEEK 4: SUGAR & SALT

Cutting out sugar is one of the most important steps of the programme. A lot of people find it really tough, but if you've got this far in the book you'll understand why it's a smart move.

The good news is that by now you should have cut out sugary drinks. That's going to help – big time – because from now on, white sugar is out.

The best way to help curb your cravings for sweet things is by balancing your blood sugar properly. You can do this by eating a little protein with each meal and also with snacks. For example, add nuts and seeds to your morning porridge, a scoop of protein powder to your smoothie, ½ avocado or some grilled fish to your lunch. As a snack, you could have a handful of seeds with an apple, vegetables dipped in hummus, a soft-boiled egg or a Protein Bomb (see page 171). Protein is slow to digest, which means you get a trickled release of energy instead of the usual spikes and dips that sugar causes.

If your sweet tooth prevails – and if that happens, trust me, you're not alone – you should definitely try using stevia, dates, figs or maple syrup instead of white sugar (see pages 30–2). Just remember, though: maple syrup, dates and figs still contain natural sugar, so don't overdose or become dependent on them instead! Everything in moderation.

If you don't like stevia first time round, try a different brand. And remember: this phase is all about retraining your brain and tastebuds. Don't give up!

One other thing: alcohol is *loaded* with sugar. For this week, you should cut it out completely. (And for the weeks that follow, have it only in very limited quantities. Beware of the 'empty' calories alcohol contains: in other words, so many calorie bangs for so few healthy bucks.)

Sorting out your salt is more straightforward. From now on, you need to ditch the table salt and replace it with a quality salt (see page 48 for a list of healthy ones). Check out what salts your local supermarket or health store sells and pick one, or order a big bag online. Easy!

I often recommend that when people are out on the trail, they take a trail spice box with them to help flavour their food. The same goes for home, or for making packed lunches or picnics. A little bit of spice really does go a long way, and if you can train yourself to flavour your meals in this way rather than by adding loads of salt, you'll be doing your body a massive favour. So, invest in a spice rack, or top up your current spice cupboard to reduce the need for extra salt in recipes.

ENJOY THE RIDE

In life, we all have the same destination! It's our journeys that are different. And that's why the journey is more important than the destination. Enjoy the journey of getting your nutrition back on track and the goodness that it will bring with it – life will be a lot richer (and longer!) if you do.

WEEKS 5 & 6: WHEAT & GLUTEN

You're halfway there! You should feel massively proud of yourself for what you've achieved so far. Hopefully you feel absolutely fantastic, and your energy levels are increasing. That means you're ready to tackle the part of the plan that I found toughest, but which has had more beneficial effects than anything else: cutting out wheat and gluten.

By cutting out wheat and gluten, you're also automatically cutting out a large array of processed junk foods such as biscuits, cakes, croissants and other unhealthy snacks. But just cutting out bread can also 'heal' people of health problems they thought were incurable. It's difficult. But like lots of difficult pursuits, the rewards are massive. The key is finding and enjoying the alternatives.

◉ For breakfast, replace your usual toast or cereal with **smoothies**, **gluten-free pancakes**, **gluten-free muffins**, **a healthy fry-up** (page 113) or filling **porridge**. (Oats do contain minute amounts of gluten, so if you are gluten-intolerant, opt for gluten-free porridge oats.)

◉ Lunches can be as simple and filling as a baked **sweet potato** on a large bed of **salad** with a few tablespoons of **hummus**, or cooked **quinoa** mixed with **roast veggies** and some **seeds**, **nuts** and **herbs**, a filling **soup** or a **Rainbow Salad** (see page 130) with some grilled fish. These will leave you feeling much more energetic than your average lunchtime sandwich ever will.

◉ For your evening meal, check out the recipe section for some great, nutritious ideas that use lots of vegetables to fill you up far better than pasta does! (Although we do have a special spaghetti recipe: check out page 157).

◉ Gluten-free snacks can be anything from nuts, seeds, fruits, pieces of fresh coconut (whole coconuts are cheap and readily available at most supermarkets), shakes or protein smoothies. Or try any of the snack recipes on pages 169–188.

- If you really miss bread, just try the amazing gluten- and wheat-free bread recipe on page 205. You can make this either savoury or sweet, and it's really filling and satisfying. Great with soup. There are also recipes for tasty wheat-free snack crackers (page 210), wheat-free brownies (page 188), Banana Walnut Bread (page 181), and even an awesome pizza that will avoid all the gluten side effects (see page 146).

- If time is not on your side and trying out new recipes seems a chore, I totally get it. Stick with the simple ones when you are busy. If you were to make a different-tasting smoothie, rainbow salad or veg soup and stir-fry each night, you'd have a varied week of meals that are super-healthy, quick, delicious and nourishing. Save the more elaborate recipes for weekends when you have more time to experiment. If you can just push on through these two weeks, you can then take stock and see whether you really still want to go back to the empty calories of bad carbs again. I'll eat my gluten-free hat if you really want to return to feeling sluggish and bloated after you have got used to some of the amazing breads and pasta alternatives out there.

A final word. Don't panic if you're not always in a position to prepare gluten-free food. Loads of delis, lunchtime takeaway places and even supermarkets are well stocked nowadays with wheat-free, dairy-free, healthy breakfast, lunch and dinner options. Browse their menus or simply tell the staff what you do and don't want in your food and have them point you in the right direction. Read labels, scan ingredients and stay open-minded.

FRIDGE REMINDERS

Focus on the end goal always, not the short-term term pain. Write your goals down and stick them to the inside of the fridge. I have in mine the words: 'No dairy, no wheat, no sugar: I want to stay fit and trim more than I want empty calories! Explore the alternatives, Bear. Be strong!' I know it sounds corny, but it works for me. Because where do we go when we feel weak? The fridge! So be prepared.

WEEK 7: BAD OILS

You're nearly there. And now, after Weeks 5 and 6, you've got an easy one.

Hopefully you'll understand by now that bad oils do a lot of unseen damage, so now is the time to replace them with healthier alternatives.

Thankfully, most supermarkets are catching up on the healthy-oil trend and sell a decent selection of quality, organic, cold-pressed, unrefined oils such as olive and hemp oil – which are great for dressings – as well as organic raw virgin coconut oil. So you don't need to travel far for your healthy alternatives.

The recipes in this book use mostly coconut oil, because it's my absolute favourite. If you don't like the taste of coconut oil, there are a few brands that have no coconut flavour. Go to your nearest health store or do a search on Google for odourless coconut oil. Or opt for avocado oil.

If you really want to use a bit of butter on non-cheat occasions, go for a grass-fed, organic butter, or use the healthier, lactose-free alternative organic ghee.

Deep-fried snacks (think potato chips and deep-fried frozen foods) also fall under the catergory 'bad oils', as they are loaded with them. If you haven't mostly given these up already, now is the time to do so. You have already learned which healthy snacks to have instead.

STAY STRONG, BE HUMBLE

Don't get complacent and don't become a bore! Both of these can trip you up. The first danger is, just as you are beginning to crack it, you start to slip, little by little, back into old, bad habits. Remember that society, the supermarkets and most probably your wider circle of friends and family will unintentionally be out to trip you up. 'Have a biscuit.' 'Do try this cake.' 'Have another drink.' You name it. As we know, it's good to cheat perhaps once a week, but not every day. Stay strong, keep alert, only allow the food past your guard that is going to help you stay strong, lean and fit. Develop the mental strength to say no. Be proud of that strength.

And finally, don't become a bore. No one likes anyone who gets self-righteous! Let your new figure and bright complexion do the talking, and only discuss the contents of this book if asked. It is meant to be our secret!

WEEK 8: MEAT & FISH

You're on the home straight. If you've got this far, give yourself a high five. If you've struggled, that's OK too. Join the club! But it gets easier and easier as the positive habits get more and more embedded.

In the wild, I'll do whatever it takes to survive. And because survival is rarely pretty, that sometimes means eating animals at the more extreme end of the scale.

But when you're not in a survival situation, things are different. Lots of people find they are eating meat twice a day. I think that's too much. We don't need a lot of meat to get enough protein, and when we do eat it we need to focus on the right kind. See pages 59–64 for the full low-down on this.

Each week, I aim for three vegetarian days, two fish days and two meat days. Don't worry if you're not crazy about fish – but replace your fish days with vegetarian days. And don't forget: processed and farmed meats are completely out. When it comes to those, remember that nothing is what it seems! Sausages have masses of wheat in them as filler, for example. Get smart. Eat natural. By the end of this week you'll be amazed at how light you will be starting to feel.

By not eating meat every day you will also save *loads* of money. What you save, you can spend on more vegetables, seeds and nuts and on a better-quality piece of meat or fish when you do eat it. Find out which butchers or farmers in your area do honest, organic, properly raised meat and check them out on a weekend off. Meat bought in bulk is much cheaper, so stock up your freezer. Or buy an organic whole chicken (instead of pricey individual chicken breasts), roast it in the oven and use it over a couple of days.

When it comes to meat and fish, opt for quality over quantity, always.

And if you're one of those people who finds themselves in a rut of eating meat every day, check out some of the great meat-free recipes in the book. Remember there are plenty of other excellent vegetarian or even vegan cookbooks out there worth investing in if you are planning to go practically meat-free or want a larger range of recipes. The research is fun. It is just the positive nutritional principles in this book that you need to stay committed to.

A FINAL WORD

You have now completed the programme. Respect! I know, like me, that you will have discovered that you have more energy and better digestion. And you will have shed a good amount of unwanted fat for sure. Be proud of the trimmer, fitter, healthier you. It has no doubt taken some dedication and hard work, but the pay-off feels good, right? I bet you've got to know your own body and mind a little better – your pitfalls, your strengths, your weaker times of day – and hopefully through it all you have discovered some hidden abs or muscles that you might never have met before! You've probably surprised yourself by what you've achieved. These are all great, positive emotions: hard fought over, and won the long way. That is why I say respect to YOU.

It's time to make a note of all those great changes in your health that you can now see and feel, especially when looking back at the questionnaire you filled out at the beginning of the eight weeks. Write down how you look, how you feel. It will be good to remind yourself every now and again of those achievements and the feelings you had when you first started to eat lean and clean.

My call to you is this: now you have done the hard work, let's build on it. Keep to the plan. It is solid and it works. And the food and recipes taste delicious. The truth is, this isn't really an 8-week plan at all. I tricked you. But you needed tricking, admit it! The rest of your life was too big an ask eight weeks ago. But now we are here: healthier, fitter and leaner. Let's keep it this way.

The principles in this book are principles for a lifetime of great nutrition. The recipes can be improved on and expanded, for sure. That's the fun part. You now know the parameters to play within. So go and play.

I now consider you to be empowered, with all the nutritional tools you need for you and your loved ones to stay happy, healthy and fit for many adventurous years to come. Nice!

stimulants 81–5
Stir-fries 152–3
stock cubes 48
stores/larder 104
strawberries
   Strawberry cheesecake 184
   see also berries
sugar 14, 30–31, 33, 52,
   84–5, 104
   cutting out 243
sugary drinks 238
sunflower seeds 71, 72
Super-healthy sausages 113
'superfoods' 73–5
Super-lean chilli 141
supplements 76–9, 80
   sports supplements 100
sweeteners 31, 32
   see also dates; maple
     syrup; stevia
sweet potatoes 29, 87
   Fried sweet potatoes 214
   Sweet potato chips 216

T

teas 237–8
   green tea 40, 75, 83, 84
   herbal teas 40, 238
   red bush (rooibos) tea
     84, 237, 238
teff flour 53
tempeh 55
Thai curry 150
Thai stir-fry 153
thyroid conditions 36,
   44, 50, 74, 87
tofu 55
tomatoes 67, 87
   Dad's tomato sauce 213
   Tomato sauce 156
Trans-fats 3
trout 37, 63

tuna 37, 62–3
turmeric 68, 75, 79

U

ulcerative colitis 52
ulcers, stomach 84
urine 44, 46, 239

V

vegan diets 60, 63, 79
vegetable oils 34–5
vegetables 16, 35, 40, 57,
   64, 65–7
   see also specific vegetables
vegetarians 63, 64
venison 61
   Super-lean chilli 141
   Venison shepherd's
     pie 140
Vitality veg 132
vitamin supplements 44,
   76–9, 80
vitamins 23, 24, 29, 30, 33,
   36, 38, 55, 57, 58, 67, 70, 71,
   75, 79, 82, 88, 102, 242

W

walnut oil 35
walnuts 37, 70, 71
   Banana walnut bread 181
   see also Fig and pecan
     energy bars
water 43–6, 238, 239
   tap water 40, 44, 45
wheat 50, 51, 52
   cutting out 245–6
wheatgrass 94
whey 57
whey protein 28
Worcestershire sauce 51–2

X

xylitol 30

Y

yeast 49, 52
yeast flakes, nutritional
   58, 242
yerba mate 84
yoghurt
   coconut yoghurt 240
   soya yoghurt 240

Z

zinc 70, 71, 102

TRANSWORLD PUBLISHERS
61–63 Uxbridge Road, London W5 5SA
www.transworldbooks.co.uk

Transworld is part of the Penguin Random House group of companies
whose addresses can be found at global.penguinrandomhouse.com

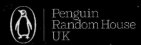
Penguin
Random House
UK

First published in Great Britain in 2015 by Bantam Press
an imprint of Transworld Publishers

A CIP catalogue record for this book
is available from the British Library.

ISBN 9780593075876

Photography by Emma Myrtle and Cristian Barnett
Food styled by Vicki Keppel-Compton and Emily Jonzen
Props by Polly Webb-Wilson
Designed and typeset in Sentinel by Smith & Gilmour
Printed in China.

Penguin Random House is committed to a sustainable
future for our business, our readers and our planet. This book
is made from Forest Stewardship Council® certified paper.

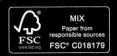

MIX
Paper from
responsible sources
FSC
www.fsc.org   FSC® C018179

13579108642